Nutrition and Aging

CURRENT CONCEPTS IN NUTRITION

Myron Winick, Editor

Institute of Human Nutrition
Columbia University College of Physicians and Surgeons

Volume 1: Nutrition and Development
Volume 2: Nutrition and Fetal Development
Volume 3: Childhood Obesity
Volume 4: Nutrition and Aging

WITHDRAWN

NUTRITION AND AGING

Edited by

MYRON WINICK

Institute of Human Nutrition
Columbia University College of Physicians and Surgeons

A WILEY-INTERSCIENCE PUBLICATION

JOHN WILEY & SONS
New York · London · Sydney · Toronto

Library of Congress Cataloging in Publication Data

Main entry under title:
Nutrition and aging.

   (Current concepts in nutrition; v. 4)
   "A Wiley-Interscience publication."
   Includes index.
   1. Aged—Nutrition. 2. Aging. 3. Nutritionally
induced diseases. I. Winick, Myron. II. Series.

RC952.5.N87   613.2'02'40565   75-34225
ISBN 0-471-95432-2

Preface

The subject of this volume, nutrition and aging, in some ways represents the result of a society that has advanced to the stage of allowing people to reach old age but that has assumed little responsibility for the care of this population. People reach old age partly because they have lived under better socioeconomic and health conditions than their forefathers. These older people have special health requirements and at the same time find themselves in economic circumstances that often preclude meeting these requirements. Thus our aged population is at increased risk of nutritional deficiency. The magnitude of this problem might best be pointed out by looking at certain statistics.

America has 20 million people who have reached what we consider to be old age. There are 22,558 nursing homes in the United States with 1.2 million beds—more nursing home beds than hospital beds. Each day more people enter "old age" than leave it. If aging is a problem, the problem is increasing, yet it is the aim of any successful society to create conditions that favor more people's reaching old age. This apparent contradiction can perhaps be best resolved by attacking the problem on two fronts: reducing the burdens that the elderly must bear and curtailing the processes that, during the early and middle years, lead to the physiological state that we at present define as old age. In a sense we must seek ways of not only slowing but actually changing the aging process as well as methods to structure the environment of those reaching old age to provide optimal health and well-being in these "twilight years." Nutrition is an important component of both of these approaches.

We are beginning to learn that nutrition during the early and middle years may be a crucial factor in determining both the rate of aging and the actual physiologic make-up of old age. This book is an attempt to examine the basic questions concerned with nutrition during earlier life and how it affects aging, and, conversely, how the process of aging affects nutritional requirements.

The book is divided into three parts:
1. Experimental models of aging.
2. Aging in normal human populations.
3. Nutrition-related diseases of old age.

Part 1 discusses the effects of aging in cultured cells. Data are presented which demonstrate that very small amounts of hydrocortisone added to the nutrient medium prolong the life of cultured cells. Thus, at least at the cellular level, hormones and nutrients interact to influence lifespan. An intriguing model of the aging placenta at the level of a complete organ system is described. Prolonging pregnancy has induced changes similar to those of the aging process. These changes are compared with changes induced by nutritional manipulations. The question being asked is, can the process of aging in this organ be accelerated by improper nutrition? This concept of "inducing" an earlier aging process by dietary manipulation is further strengthened by data relating early dietary intake in rats to subsequent longevity. The work suggests that the lifespan of laboratory animals can be either more than doubled or drastically curtailed by dietary manipulation during the growing period. The investigators have concluded that if dietary intervention is to have a beneficial effect on the diseases of age and the span of life, it must be done early in life.

In essence then, a number of basic studies are suggesting that the process of aging is in part programmed early in life and that nutrition may be an important factor in writing this program.

In Part 2, two chapters outline the normal physiologic and metabolic changes of old age and how these changes make older people susceptible to certain diseases. In addition, they discuss what we already know about the protein and amino acid requirements of the elderly. The data suggest that because of normally occurring changes, the older individual develops specific nutrient requirements that were not present before.

Chapter 6 addresses itself to the actual feeding problems encountered by the elderly. Data on food preferences and nutritional status in elderly citizens of middle Tennessee are presented as a skeleton for general discussion of feeding programs. For example the Tennessee survey notes that breakfast is eaten by 90% of the elderly and that 37% consider it their favorite meal. Should we have more breakfast programs? If so, how should they be organized? Old people eat more frequently. Should we develop nutritious snack foods? Are iron and calcium supplements desirable? All of these and other questions are discussed.

Thus nutrition influences the aging process and aging influences the nutritional requirements. Faulty nutrition anywhere in this cycle has undesirable consequences.

Part 3 discusses some of the more common and more serious diseases of old age that are in part related to nutrition. Two diseases related to calcium and phosphorus intake, osteoporosis and peridontal disease, which results in loss of teeth, are discussed. Although both areas are still somewhat controversial, the investigators conclude that increased calcium and reduced phosphorus in the diet may slow both of these processes which involve bone resorption, that osteoporosis is best treated with a combination of fluoride and calcium, and that peridontal disease can be reversed on high calcium intakes. Next the role of fiber in the diet is reviewed. Again all of the data are not in, but there is a strong suggestion that our low fiber diet, which accompanies affluence, is contributing to the high incidence of diverticular disease and cancer of the colon. The author concludes that

> "... many will recall an era of interest in vegetarianism and a wide enthusiasm for whole grain cereals and bran supplements, which had its peak over forty years ago. There now appears to be a more convincing but still incomplete rationale for regulation of vegetable fiber intake, with some prospects of prevention of morbidity from colonic disease in an aging population."

Finally, obesity and atherosclerosis are discussed. Data are presented which demonstrate that both intrinsic aging processes and environmental factors operative over many years apparently act in concert with unknown genetic factors to produce metabolic changes in carbohydrate and lipid metabolism resulting in highly prevalent age-related diseases, such as diabetes and atherosclerosis. The most prominent environmental factor may well be excessive caloric intake during adult life.

Although this book cannot cover all of the relationships between nutrition and aging, it does attempt to develop the basic thesis that aging is a process that occurs over a lifetime and that how we eat during that lifetime will in part determine how fast we age and what "diseases of the elderly" we contract. In addition, just being old changes our metabolism, our appetite, our whole body physiology, and of necessity our nutritional requirements. New approaches to feeding the elderly must be devised. At this time the book may raise more questions than it answers. That is the nature of science. However, since the well-being of at least 20 million Americans is involved, it is hoped that the reader will emerge not only better informed but better able to deal with those problems which can be dealt with and better able to begin to wrestle with the more difficult problems which desperately await creative solutions.

MYRON WINICK

New York, New York
January 1976

Contents

Nutrition and Aging

PART 1

Experimental Models of Aging

1

A Model System Approach
to the Biology of Aging

V. J. CRISTOFALO

The Wistar Institute of Anatomy and Biology,
Philadelphia, Pennsylvania

INTRODUCTION

It is now reasonably well established that populations of normal diploid human fibroblasts can proliferate in culture for only limited periods of time. Typically, after explantation, there is a period of rapid proliferation when the cultures can be subcultivated relatively often, followed by a period of declining proliferative capacity during which the cells become granular, debris accumulates, and ultimately the culture is lost. The work of Swim and Parker (1) and Hayflick and Moorhead (2) establishes the generality of this phenomenon.

Figure 1 shows the typical lifespan of a culture of human fetal lung cells. After the period of rapid growth (about 150 days under these conditions), there is a declining proliferative rate and the culture is eventually lost. A similar limitation on the growth of chick cells has been noted by several authors (3, 4). During the last 14 years, in many laboratories throughout the world, these findings have been duplicated not only for human cells, but for cells from other species as well (4, 5). The doubling capacities of various populations of cells in culture are reproducible within relatively narrow limits. For example, about 50 population doublings occur with human embryonic fibroblasts, while embryonic chick fibroblasts have a doubling potential of about 25 passages.

This work was supported by grants HDO2721 and HDO6323 from the National Institute of Child Health and Human Development.

3

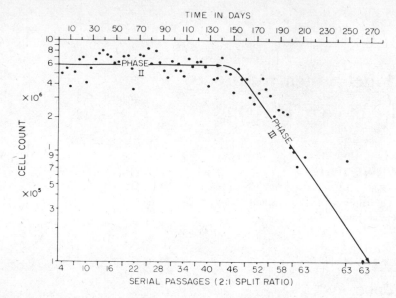

Figure 1. Cell counts determined at each passage of human diploid cell, strain WI-44. The initial plateau during phase II, with no apparent loss of biological function as measured by constant doubling time, is followed by phase III, where doubling time increases exponentially. (From (6). Reprinted with permission of Academic Press, New York.)

Hence the notion that isolated animal cells are capable of unlimited proliferation in culture, as proposed by Carrel and his co-workers (7, 8), does not appear to be the case, except where spontaneous transformation occurs giving rise to cultures that maintain their proliferative capacity for what seems to be indefinite periods of time. The propensity for spontaneous transformation varies among species. Human and chick fibroblast cultures almost never transform spontaneously whereas rodent cells often do. In addition, certain cultures derived from human lymphoid elements seem to retain the normal diploid karyotype and have an indefinite lifespan (9, 10). However, none of these appears to meet the full criteria of being karyologically normal.

Initially the inability of untransformed cell cultures to proliferate indefinitely was ascribed to various technical difficulties, such as inadequate nutrition, pH variation, toxic metabolic products, and microcontaminants. However, in an extensive series of experiments, Hayflick and Moorhead (2) showed that clonal degeneration was unrelated, at least in any simple, direct way, to any of these factors. When mixtures of young and old populations (male and female), distinguishable by karyotypic markers (Barr bodies), were grown in the same pool of medium, the older population was lost after it had undergone a total of approximately 50 population doublings, while the younger population continued to proliferate until its 50 or so expected doublings had been completed. Such results would seem to rule out any direct effect of the composition of the medium, or the presence of contaminating microorganisms or toxic end products of metabolism.

Loss of proliferative capacity cannot be related to depletion of some essential, nonreplicating metabolite, since the initial presence of 2^{50} molecules of even the lightest element, hydrogen, would have a mass in excess of that of a single cell. Hayflick and Moorhead (2) and Hayflick (6) concluded from these data that the limited lifespan phenomenon must be intrinsic to the cell, and they interpreted their observations as a cellular expression of senescence.

The suggestion that aging changes are reflected in various properties of tissue cultures is not new. For example, it has long been known that age-associated changes that occur in plasma can inhibit cell growth *in vitro* (11). In addition, the time elapsing prior to cell migration from explanted tissue fragments increases with increasing age (12, 13, 14). These are both examples of the expression, *in vitro,* of aging *in vivo.* The studies of Hayflick and Moorhead (2) and Hayflick (6) focus attention on the occurrence of senescence *in vitro.*

To one interested in the study of senescence, the important questions are the following: *(1)* Does aging *in vitro* bear any relationship to aging of the whole organism? *(2)* Do studies carried out in cell culture have any relevance to aging in the whole animal? In approaching these questions one must remember that it is very difficult with our present state of knowledge to pinpoint what relationship, if any, exists between aging *in vivo* and aging *in vitro.*

On one hand, it is reasonably well documented for some populations of proliferating cells that, after an initial period of rapid cell division, there is a decline in the proliferative capacity as the animal ages (15, 16). Buetow (16) has recently tabulated and reviewed the literature on age-associated changes in cellular proliferation rates. In general, there is a decline in mitotic activity in a wide variety of tissues of humans and various rodent species. More recently Lesher and Sacher (17), Thrasher (18), and Cameron (19, 20) have confirmed these reports in detailed studies with mouse tissues.

Another group of studies which bears on this point involves the serial transplantation of normal somatic tissues to new, young inbred hosts each time the current recipient approaches old age. For example, the work of Daniel and co-workers (21) in which mouse mammary glands were transplanted into gland-free mammary fat pads of young, isogenic female mice, shows that the growth rate of a normal gland declines with time. Thus the normal mammary gland has a limited ability to proliferate *in vivo* even under these most favorable growth conditions. Similar findings have been published for transplanted skin (22, 23) and for bone marrow cells (24, 25). Hence, in general, normal cells serially transplanted to inbred hosts seem to show a decline in proliferative capacity and probably cannot survive indefinitely.

In addition, age-associated declines in proliferative capacity have been documented for isoproterenol-stimulated salivary gland (26), and for elements of the mouse immune system (27, 28). Thus, a decline in proliferative capacity represents one more kind of gradual functional failure that occurs in the aging animal.

Perhaps the most striking line of evidence for the relationship of a limited lifespan *in vitro* to aging *in situ* springs from a variety of works which suggest a cumulative effect of *in situ* plus *in vitro* aging by showing a relationship between the age of the cell donor and the proliferative capacity of the cells derived from that donor. For example, Hayflick (6) found a dramatic difference between cell lines derived from human embryo and human adult lung. In addition, Goldstein and his co-workers (29) found that an inverse correlation existed between the age of the donor and the number of population doublings that a series of skin cultures could achieve.

Martin and co-workers (30) carried out an extensive study in which over 100 mass cultures of fibroblastlike human diploid cells from a variety of donors varying in age from newborn to 90 years were used. They found a significant regression of growth potential as a function of the age of the donor.

Goldstein (29) and Martin (30) and their co-workers have shown that cells from patients with progeria or with Werner's syndrome (both diseases associated with premature aging) have a reduced proliferative capacity as compared with cells from normal (control) donors of the same ages. In addition, cells derived from diabetic individuals, who often show at an earlier chronological age some of the degenerative changes associated with aging, have a reduced ability to grow and survive in culture, as manifested by a reduced plating efficiency (29).

We are not, of course, suggesting that animals die because they exhaust the supply of, for example, lung fibroblasts, bone marrow, or skin cells. In fact, as in the *in vivo* studies of Daniel and others described above, it is impossible to directly relate the time course of this loss of proliferative capacity *in vitro* to the lifespan of the animal, since in some cases the transplant has a longer lifespan than that of the animal from which it was derived (23). On the other hand, it seems reasonable to expect that the study of the regulation of cell proliferation *in vitro* would lend important insight into the mechanism of regulation of cell proliferation *in vivo* and its ramifications for aging in the intact animal. In addition, it is not clear whether, in any case, a reduced rate of proliferation would ordinarily result in any survival-compromising shortage of cells. It is possible, however, that failure in the regulation of proliferative capacity could be accompanied by failures in other cellular functions that would then compromise the ability of the animal to respond adaptively to a changing environment.

Perhaps one of the best documented physiological changes that occur during cellular aging *in vitro* is a marked increase in lysosomes and lysosomal enzymes. The lysosomes appear to be involved in a variety of degenerative processes including, for example, autolysis during inflammatory reactions, as well as programmed involutional changes, such as the resorption of the tadpole's tail. Allison and Paton (31) have reported that the lysosomes of WI-38 cells contain a DNA depolymerase that can cause chromosomal breaks and, since it has two active sites, can destroy both strands of DNA with a single hit.

Previous work in our laboratory on acid phosphatase and β glucuronidase activities in crude homogenates of human diploid cell cultures showed an increase in the specific activity of these enzymes during *in vitro* aging (32). These enzymes are typically marker enzymes for lysosomes, and we concluded from these findings that older cells contained more lysosomes. Since then, this conclusion has been further documented in electron microscopic studies both from our laboratory (33) and by others (34, 35).

Based on these findings, several years ago we initiated a series of experiments designed to further our understanding of the role of lysosomes in cellular aging *in vitro*. These included studies on the subcellular distribution of lysosomal enzymes, the fraction of activity that was membrane bound, and the action of a known lysosome stabilizer, hydrocortisone, on these parameters (36, 37).

Hydrocortisone (cortisol), at a concentration of 5 μg/ml, did retard leakage of acid phosphatase from crude lysosomal preparations (38); however, the most striking result of these studies was the increase in lifespan of the cultures in the presence of 5 μg/ml hydrocortisone (14 μM) (37-39). Macieira-Coelho (40) had reported a similar finding for human cells treated with cortisone.

This hydrocortisone effect on cell lifespan represents the action of a chemically defined modulator of cell division and population lifespan, and we have further documented these observations in the hope of using hydrocortisone as a probe for modulating the regulation of cell division and the limitation of proliferative capacity of these diploid cell cultures (37-39, 41).

As a result of our preliminary studies, the principal features of the hydrocortisone effect can be summarized as follows: *(1)* Replicate experiments based on cell counts have shown that the lifespan in terms of actual population doublings was extended 30 to 40% by the continuous inclusion of 5 μg/ml hydrocortisone in the medium. *(2)* This effect seemed to be maximal with 5 μg/ml hydrocortisone. *(3)* There was no rescue with the hormone. Once a culture had reached the stage where it could no longer achieve confluency, hydrocortisone would not reverse this condition. *(4)* If hydrocortisone was added at different periods in the lifespan, the magnitude of the lifespan extension was in direct proportion to the amount of time the culture was grown in the presence of the hormone. *(5)* The saturation density of the culture was increased in the presence of the hormone. *(6)* The over-all effect on proliferative capacity was not due to increased plating efficiency or improved adhesion to the glass or plastic surface.

Since these effects of hydrocortisone represent modulation of cell lifespan by a chemically defined probe, we have pursued these studies in the hope of better understanding the mechanism by which cell lifespan is regulated.

MATERIALS AND METHODS

Except where noted, all studies were done with human diploid cell lines WI-38 and WI-26 (2, 6). These were obtained either from frozen stock maintained here at the Wistar Institute or from Dr. Leonard Hayflick of Stanford University. The cells were grown as previously described (42) in autoclavable Eagle's MEM (Auto-Pow, Flow Laboratories, Rockville, Md.) modified by the addition of Eagle's BME vitamins. Immediately before use, the medium was supplemented with L-glutamine (2 mmole), NaHCO₃ (20 mmole), and fetal calf serum (10% v/v). Cultures were grown at 37°C in an atmosphere of 5% CO_2 and 95% air, and were monitored for mycoplasma by the method of Levine (43).

Routine subcultivations were carried out when monolayers were confluent. The cells were released from the glass by treatment with trypsin (0.25%) in Ca^{2+}- and Mg^{2+}-free phosphate buffered saline solution. After suspension in medium containing 10% fetal calf serum, the cells were counted and inoculated into appropriate vessels at a density of 1×10^4 cells/cm².

Cell population doublings were calculated by comparison of the cell counts per vessel at seeding and when the cultures reached confluency. All cell counts were done electronically using a Coulter Counter. Autoradiography was carried out by our standard procedures (42) in which tritiated thymidine (^{3}H-dT) was added to the culture to a final concentration of 0.1 μCi/ml (specific activity 2 Ci/mmole).

For liquid scintillation counting, coverslips were prepared as for autoradiography, removed at appropriate intervals, dipped in cold 10% trichloroacetic acid, and placed directly into scintillation vials and counted in an Intertechnique Liquid Scintillation Spectrometer.

For evaluation of the effect of various steroids on DNA synthesis, the hormones were purchased from commercial suppliers at the best grade of purity available. Active hormones were also checked for the presence of impurities by standard thin-layer chromatographic methods. For autoradiographic analysis of their biological activity the conditions used were identical with those reported previously. All hormones were used at a concentration of 5 μg/ml. Where solubility was limiting, the hormones were dissolved in 100% ethanol. Subsequent dilution was carried out in medium to give a final concentration of ethanol of no more than 0.5%. Paired controls were always run with an identical concentration of ethanol in the medium. For all active hormones the change in the labeling index was correlated with direct cell counts.

RESULTS

Initially, our studies were designed to determine how the effect of hydrocortisone in extending lifespan was expressed during a single population growth cycle. Figure 2 shows the results of a typical growth curve in which cell number, DNA synthesis determined chemically, and radioactivity incorporated into DNA from ^{3}H-dT were monitored for hydrocortisone-treated and control cells. The zero time point on the figure represents 24 hours after seeding both cultures with identical cell numbers. During the growth cycle the curves diverged, and by 72 hours there was a clear and consistent difference between the treated and control cultures. The DNA content of the culture followed the same pattern, with the hormone-treated cultures having a higher rate of DNA synthesis. Finally, the kinetics of radioactivity incorporated into DNA from the ^{3}H-dT precursor paralleled the rate of synthesis of DNA. Thus, ^{3}H-dT would seem to be an appropriate probe to follow the hydrocortisone effect on cell proliferation.

In studies reported elsewhere (44, 45) we have shown that the ki-

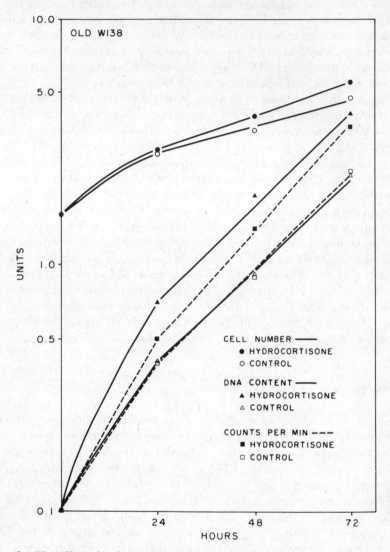

Figure 2. The effect of hydrocortisone on cell proliferation, DNA synthesis, and ³H-dT incorporated into DNA in logarithmically growing WI-38 cultures (passage 42). (From (45). Reprinted with permission of Plenum Press, New York.)

netics of thymidine uptake and phosphorylation were not significantly affected by the presence of the hydrocortisone. However, these studies, although establishing the effects of hydrocortisone directly on DNA synthesis rather than on ^{3}H-dT metabolism, really are directed at the population level. Since there is an exponential decline with age in the fraction of cycling cells, it was of interest to determine whether the addition of hydrocortisone increased this fraction.

Table 1 shows the effect, in terms of nuclear labeling, of treatment of previously untreated older cells for 24 or 48 hours with hydrocor-

Table 1 The Effect of Length of Exposure to Hydrocortisone on the Incorporation of ^{3}H-dT by Young and Old WI-38 Cells[a]

Treatment	Exposure (hours)	Percent labeled nuclei	
		Young	Old
None	24	41.5 ± 6.6 (5)	38.6 ± 10.3 (3)
	48	79.8 ± 5.7 (6)[b]	45.9 ± 3.4 (15)[c]
Hydrocortisone	24	60.0 ± 6.5 (5)	50.0 ± 10.2 (3)
	48	92.3 ± 1.9 (6)[b]	64.6 ± 4.1 (14)[c]

[a] Mean ± standard error of mean. Numbers in parentheses indicate number of samples.
[b] p < .005.
[c] p < .001.

tisone. For these studies, hydrocortisone was present for either 24 or 48 hours while the ^{3}H-dT was present for the standard period. There was a statistically significant increase in the percentage of cells in both young and old cultures incorporating ^{3}H-dT in the presence of hydrocortisone after 48 hours. Here the effect is much more striking in older cultures, where the increase in the presence of the hormone was about 45%, whereas in young cultures it was only about 15%. Parallel cultures showed an increase in cell number in the presence of the hormone and the results are consistent with stimulation of both DNA synthesis and cell division.

Hence the hydrocortisone-mediated increase in DNA synthesis seems to be due, in part at least, to an increase in the fraction of cells in the proliferating pool. Hydrocortisone appears to amplify the stimulus for proliferation.

To evaluate the effect of hydrocortisone on DNA synthesis, experiments were designed to determine whether or not the biological activity was specific for the molecular structure of hydrocortisone. Various steroids were assayed for their biological activity with WI-38 cells as determined by the increase in the percentage of labeled nuclei in the culture. The compounds tested fell into three groups: those that were very active, hydrocortisone being the most active in stimulating DNA synthesis; those that were clearly inhibitory to DNA synthesis, testosterone being the most inhibitory; and a third group in which there may have been moderate borderline effects but which were not significantly different from the control.

Figure 3 shows a comparison of the molecular structures of hydrocortisone and the other five stimulatory steroids. Note that all have the 3 keto, Δ4 configuration in Ring A, an 11β-hydroxy group, and a keto group at C-20. Other functional groups such as the 17α and the

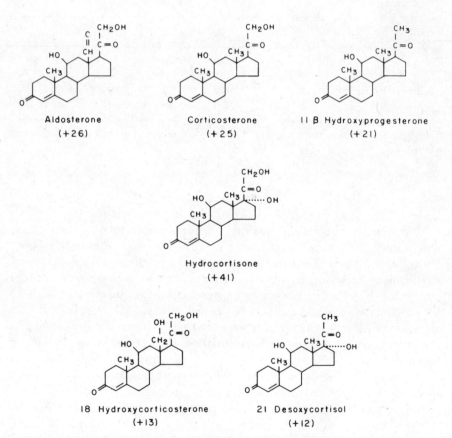

Figure 3. Molecular structures of steroids active in stimulating DNA synthesis. (From (45). Reprinted with permission of Plenum Press, New York.)

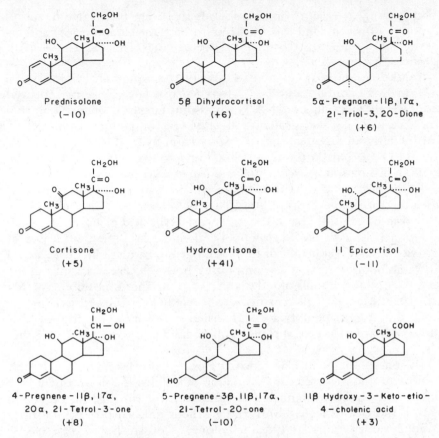

Prednisolone
(−10)

5β Dihydrocortisol
(+6)

5α- Pregnane -11β,17α,
21-Triol-3, 20-Dione
(+6)

Cortisone
(+5)

Hydrocortisone
(+41)

11 Epicortisol
(−11)

4-Pregnene -11β, 17α,
20α, 21-Tetrol-3-one
(+8)

5-Pregnene -3β,11β,17α,
21-Tetrol-20-one
(−10)

11β Hydroxy -3-Keto-etio-
4-cholenic acid
(+3)

Figure 4. Molecular structures of steroids in which key functional groups have been changed. (From (45). Reprinted with permission of Plenum Press, New York.)

21-hydroxy groups, present in hydrocortisone but not in some of the others, or the C-18 methyl group, present in all but aldosterone and 19-hydroxycorticosterone, seemed of minor and variable significance to the action of the hormone.

Figure 4 shows the results of experiments designed to test the effect of variations in these three functional groups on the biological activity of these hormones. The first row are examples of variations in the structure of the A ring. Prednisolone, which has a structure identical with hydrocortisone except for one additional double bond in the A ring, was a mild inhibitor of DNA synthesis. Similar synthetic steroids, such as dexamethasone and triamcinolone (not shown), are either inhibitory or without effect on DNA synthesis. Reduction of the double bond in ring A resulted in compounds that were ineffective in stimulating cell division, and this was true for both the cis and trans configurations (5β-dihydrocortisol and 5α-pregnane-11β,17α,21-triol-3,20-dione, respectively).

In the second row of Fig. 4 are two compounds in which the 11β-hydroxy configuration was altered. Cortisone (11 keto) appeared consistently to stimulate DNA synthesis but to such a small extent that the data were not statistically significant. The compound 11-epicortisol, an inhibitor of DNA synthesis, differs from hydrocortisone in having the 11-OH group in the α position. Thus, the recognition sites in the cell can distinguish between 11α- and β-hydroxy steroids.

In the last row are compounds in which reduction of the C-20 keto group (4-pregnane-11β,17α,20α,21-tetrol-3-one) caused loss of activity. Removal of the side chain, leaving a carboxylic acid group in the C-20 position (11β-hydroxy-3-keto-etio-4-cholenic acid), also caused loss of activity. Finally, reduction of the 3 keto group resulted in a compound with inhibitory effects. This compound, however, also has a shift in the position of the double bond from the 4 to the 5 position, so that interpretation of this result is not clear. Cortol (5β-pregnane-3α,11β,17,20α,21-pentol), a 3-OH structure in which both the A and B rings are saturated (not shown), is also a mild inhibitor of DNA synthesis.

In general the molecular specificity of hydrocortisone activity is very similar to that reported for stimulation of cell division in confluent 3T3 mouse fibroblasts by Thrash and Cunningham (46). The major exception is the lack of activity with the synthetic glucocorticoids, prednisolone, dexamethasone, and triamcinolone, all of which were effective in the mouse system but not in the human system. We have compared the effects of these three hormones over concentrations ranging from 5×10^{-3} μg/ml to 100 μg/ml. None was stimulating. In fact at the highest concentrations they were slightly inhibitory.

Still to be explained is the requirement for activity of hydrocortisone concentrations on the order of several hundredfold higher than that found in circulating human blood. The higher concentration required for response may reflect the absence or low level of specific cytosol receptors for hydrocortisone. Croce and co-workers (47) have reported that cytosol receptors for glucocorticoids are very low or absent in WI-38 cells. Perhaps the differences in responsiveness of various tissues *in vivo* and *in vitro* are concentration-dependent. When high-affinity cytosol receptors are present very low concentrations might elicit a response. Alternatively, cells without such receptors might be unresponsive to a given hormone; however, if the concentration was raised to a high enough level, then the interaction of the hormone with its target could occur. We are currently studying the nature and subcellular localization of specific protein receptors for hydrocortisone in young and old cells.

We have established that this effect of hydrocortisone on the stimulation of cell proliferation is highly specific for human diploid fibroblastlike cells (44, 45), and that the inhibitory effect previously observed occurs with permanently proliferating cell lines with an indefinite lifespan. Since the loss of proliferative capacity in these diploid populations has been shown to be due to an exponential increase in the number of noncycling or very slowly cycling cells in the population (42), it was of interest to determine if cultures grown continuously in the presence of hydrocortisone showed the same heterogeneity.

Figure 5 shows the percentage of labeled nuclei as a function of cumulative number of population doublings (determined by direct cell count) at each subcultivation over the lifespan of the culture. Both female-derived (WI-38) and male-derived (WI-26) cell cultures were studied. The control and hormone-treated cultures were started together. Initially, nearly 100% of the cells were labeled in both cases. As the lifespan progressed, however, the accelerated rate of proliferation of the hormone-treated population was shown by the more rapid traverse of the clear bars (representing the hormone-treated cultures) across the abscissa; i.e., the hormone-treated cultures were doubling more rapidly.

The decline in the fraction of labeled cells was more rapid in the control cultures and they phased out well before the hydrocortisone-treated cultures; however, the pattern of decline in labeling was the same in both cases. Hydrocortisone seemed to retain the cells in the actively proliferating pool for longer periods.

Finally, it is important to note that, just as with the short-term autoradiographic experiment, the differences between hydrocortisone-treated and control cultures were greater as the culture aged. However, in both cultures the percentage of cells responding to the stimulus for division declined with age. The rate of decline was slower in the hydrocortisone-treated culture. Thus it appears from these experiments as well that the hydrocortisone is amplifying the primary signal for division. Further evidence for this interpretation is provided in Fig. 6. Here, in the absence of serum there was essentially no division; the primary signal for division was clearly serum. With graded increases in serum there was a graded response in the fraction of cells incorporating labeled precursor. Note that in the presence of hydrocortisone, 0.3% serum gave a response higher than 10% serum without

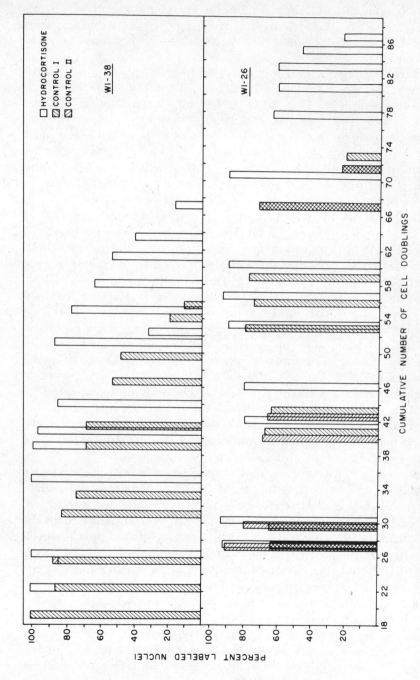

Figure 5. The effect of hydrocortisone on the fraction of labeled nuclei in the culture after 30 hours exposure to ³H-dT at intervals throughout the lifespan of both WI-38 and WI-26 cells. (From (45). Reprinted with permission of Plenum Press, New York.)

16

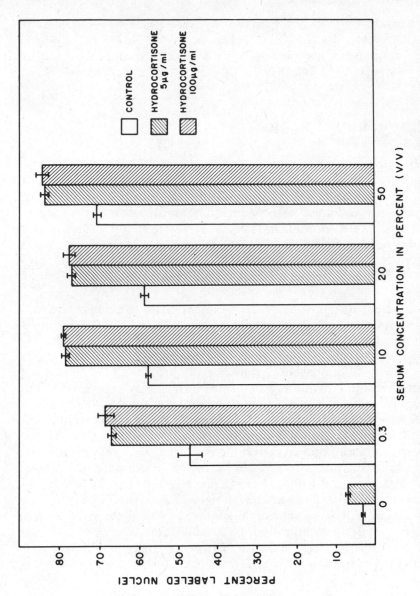

Figure 6. The effect of serum concentration and hydrocortisone on nuclear labeling in WI-38 cultures. (From (45). Reprinted with permission of Plenum Press, New York.)

hydrocortisone, and 10% serum plus hydrocortisone was equivalent to or greater than 50% serum. Similar amplifying effects were found when serum and hydrocortisone were added to confluent, contact-inhibited monolayers of WI-38 cells (45).

DISCUSSION AND SUMMARY

The data presented above show the following. (1) The extension of the lifespan of human diploid cells by hydrocortisone is due, in part at least, to an increase of the fraction of cells synthesizing DNA. We have not ruled out additional effects, including an increase in the rate of transit of the cells through the various cell cycle periods. This is currently being investigated. (2) The effect on cell division, however, is not mediated through changes in thymidine metabolism alone. (3) Hydrocortisone appears to amplify the serum stimulus for division.

We have also shown that the stimulatory effect of hydrocortisone on DNA synthesis is highly specific for human diploid fibroblastlike cells (44, 45) and for certain molecular configurations in the substituted steroid nucleus. The recognition sites require unsaturation at the 4-5 position in ring A, the keto group at position 3, the 11β-hydroxy group, and an additional keto group at position 20.

Hydrocortisone, cortisone, and corticosteroids have been reported to prolong the *in vitro* survival time of several cell types (48-50). These studies have been concerned with postmitotic maintenance of the cultures. Macieira-Coelho (40), however, was the first to report the increase in proliferative lifespan of diploid, fibroblastlike cells in culture.

Division-stimulating effects with hydrocortisone have also been reported by Castor and Prince (51) for cartilage cells and by Smith and co-workers (52) for human fetal lung cells. Recently, Thrash and Cunningham (53) have shown the stimulation of division by hydrocortisone in density inhibited 3T3 cells, and Armelin (54) and Gospodarowicz (55) have shown that hydrocortisone amplifies the activity of the pituitary- and brain-derived polypeptides that stimulate cell division.

In considering possible ways to explain these results we must remember that although changes in transcription represent the best-defined action of glucocorticoids, there is a wide range of other less well understood effects of steroids, many of them involving various membrane effects.

Perhaps the most difficult assignment is to propose a model in which despite the continual presence of hydrocortisone that stimulates cell proliferation and prolongs cell lifespan, the population is still lost. A summary of some possibilities for such a model is presented in Fig. 7.

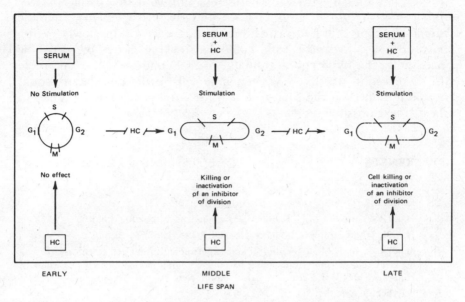

Figure 7. Possible effects of hydrocortisone on human diploid fibroblastlike cultures. (From (45). Reprinted with permission of Plenum Press, New York.)

Aging of the population is reflected at the cellular level by a transition from a rapidly cycling state to one or a series of more slowly cycling states, and finally to a sterile state, that is, a state in which the cells are arrested or are cycling so slowly as to be unable to repopulate the culture vessel. These three transitions are shown in the center portion of Fig. 7. One simple interpretation of the data is that the steroid delays these transitions.

Another possible interpretation is shown in the upper portion of the figure and is based by analogy on the work of Bresciani (56), in which he showed that as mammary cells differentiate, they lose responsiveness to one hormone but acquire or maintain responsiveness to other hormonal stimuli. Possibly young cells are responsive to 10% serum initially, but eventually lose their responsiveness to this concentration of serum and undergo a transition to a second state where 10% serum plus hydrocortisone is required to elicit a division response. Alternatively, there may be a second population in the culture which succeeds the first and which will only proliferate in the presence of serum plus hydrocortisone.

Finally, a third possibility is shown in the lower portion of the figure and presupposes that slowly cycling or arrested cells inhibit the growth of cells that are capable of division either simply by occupying space or by eliciting an inhibitor or chalone into the environment. In these rapidly dividing cells hydrocortisone has no effect. In the slowly cycling cells, however, hydrocortisone could be working either by somehow inactivating the hypothetical inhibitor or by killing the cells responsible for its secretion. In this way, the young cells in the population would not be inhibited to the same extent. Our current work is designed to clarify these possibilities.

REFERENCES

1. Swim, H. E., and Parker, R. F. *Am. J. Hyg.* **66:**235 (1957).
2. Hayflick, L. and Moorhead, P. S. *Exp. Cell Res.* **25:**585 (1961).
3. Haff, R. F. and Swim, H. E. *Proc. Soc. Exp. Biol. Med.* **93:**200 (1956).
4. Hay, R. J. and Strehler, B. L. *Exp. Gerontol.* **2:**123 (1967).
5. Simons, J. W. I. M. A theoretical and experimental approach to the relationship between cell variability and aging *in vitro.* In *Aging in Cell and Tissue Culture.* E. Holečkovà and V. J. Cristofalo, Eds. Plenum, New York, 1970, pp. 25-39.
6. Hayflick, L. *Exp. Cell Res.* **37:**614 (1965).
7. Ebeling, A. H. *J. Exp. Med.* **17:**273 (1913).
8. Ebeling, A. H. *J. Exp. Med.* **34:**231 (1921).
9. Moore, G. E. and McLimans, W. F. *J. Theoret. Biol.* **20:**217 (1968).
10. Levy, J. A., Virolainen, M., and Defendi, V. *Cancer* **22:**517 (1968).
11. Carrel, A. and Ebeling, A. H. *J. Exp. Med.* **34:**599 (1921).
12. Carrel, A. and Burrows, M. T. *J. A. M. A.* **55:**1379 (1910).
13. Carrel, A. and Burrows, M. T. *J. A. M. A.* **55:**1554 (1910).
14. Carrel, A. and Burrows, M. T. *J. Exp. Med.* **13:**562 (1911).
15. LeBlond, C. P. *Classification of cell populations on the basis of their proliferative behavior.* National Cancer Institute Monograph No. 14. C. C. Congdon and P. Mori-Chavez, Eds. 1964, pp. 119–145.
16. Buetow, D. E. Cellular content and cellular proliferation changes in the tissues and organs of the aging mammal. In *Cellular and Molecular Renewal in the Mammalian Body.* I. L. Cameron and J. O. Thrasher, Eds., Academic, New York, 1971, pp. 87–104.
17. Lesher, S. and Sacher, G. A. *Exp. Gerontol.* **3:**211 (1968).
18. Thrasher, J. O. *Exp. Gerontol.* **6:**19 (1971).
19. Cameron, I. L. *J. Gerontol.* **27:**157 (1972).
20. Cameron, I. L. *J. Gerontol.* **27:**162 (1972).
21. Daniel, C. W., DeOme, K. B., Young, J. T., Blair, P. B. and Faulkin, L. J. *Proc. Nat. Acad. Sci.* **61:**53 (1968).
22. Krohn, P. L. *Proc. Roy. Soc. Med.* **157:**128 (1962).

23. Krohn, P. L. Transplantation and aging. In *Topics of the Biology of Aging*. P. L. Krohn, Ed. Interscience, New York, 1966, pp. 159–162.

24. Siminovitch, L., Till, J. E., and McCulloch, E. A. *J. Cell. Comp. Physiol.* **64:**23 (1964).

25. Cudkowicz, G., Upton, A. C., Shearer, G. M. and Hughes, W. L. *Nature* **201:**165 (1964).

26. Adelman, R. C., Stein, G., Roth, G. S. and Englander, D. *Mech. Ag. Develop.* **1:**49 (1972).

27. Price, G. B. and Makinodan, T. *J. Immunol.* **108:**403 (1972).

28. Price, G. B. and Makinodan, T. *J. Immunol.* **108:**413 (1972).

29. Goldstein, S., Littlefield, J. W. and Soeldner, J. S. *Proc. Nat. Acad. Sci.* **64:**155 (1969).

30. Martin, G. M., Sprague, C. A. and Epstein, C. J. *Lab. Invest.* **23:**86 (1970).

31. Allison, A. C. and Paton, G. R. *Nature* (London) **207:**1170 (1965).

32. Cristofalo, V. J., Parris, N. and Kritchevsky, D. *J. Cell Physiol.* **69:**263 (1967).

33. Lipetz, J. and Cristofalo, V. J. *J. Ultrastruc. Res.* **39:**43 (1972).

34. Robbins, E., Levine E. M. and Eagle, H. *J. Exp. Med.* **131:**1211 (1970).

35. Brandes, D., Murphy, D. G., Anton, E. and Barnard S. *J. Ultrastruc. Res.* **39:**465 (1972).

36. Cristofalo, V. J., Kabakjian, J. R. and Kritchevsky, D. *Proc. Soc. Exp. Biol. Med.* **126:**649 (1967).

37. Cristofalo, V. J. Metabolic aspects of aging in diploid human cells. In *Aging in Cell and Tissue Culture*. E. Holečkovà and V. J. Cristofalo, Eds., Plenum, New York, 1970, pp. 83–119.

38. Cristofalo, V. J. and Kabakjian, J. R. *Mech. Aging and Develop.* (In press).

39. Cristofalo, V. J. *Proc. Eighth Inter. Cong. Gerontol.* **II:** 6 (1969).

40. Macieira-Coelho, A. *Experientia* **22:**390 (1966).

41. Cristofalo, V. J., Kobler, D., Kabakjian, J., Mackessy, J. and Baker, B. *In Vitro* **6:**396 (1971).

42. Cristofalo, V. J. and Sharf, B. B. *Exp. Cell Res.* **76:**419 (1973).

43. Levine, E. M. *Exp. Cell Res.* **74:**99 (1972).

44. Cristofalo, V. J. Cellular senescence: Factors modulating cell proliferation *in vitro*. In *Molecular and Cellular Mechanisms of Aging*. F. Bourlière, Y. Courtois, A. Macieira-Coelho and L. Roberts, Eds. Volume 27, INSERM, Paris, 1974, pp. 65–92.

45. Cristofalo, V. J. The effect of hydrocortisone on DNA synthesis and cell division during aging *in vitro*. In *Impairment of Cellular Functions During Aging and Development*. V. J. Cristofalo and E. Holečkovà, Eds. Plenum New York, 1975, pp. 7–22.

46. Thrash C. R., Ho. T. and Cunningham, D. D. *J. Biol. Chem.* **249:**6099 (1974).

47. Croce, C. M., Litwack, G., and Koprowski, H. *Proc. Nat. Acad. Sci.* **70:**1268 (1973).

48. Arpels, C., Babcock, V. J. and Southam, C. M. *Proc. Soc. Exp. Biol. Med.* **115:**102 (1964).

49. Yuan, G. C. and Chang, R. S. *Proc. Soc. Exp. Biol. Med.* **130:**934 (1969).

50. Yuan G. C., Chang, R. S., Little, J. B. and Cornil, G. *J. Gerontol.* **22:**174 (1967).

51. Castor, C. W. and Prince, R. K. *Biochim. Biophys. Acta* **83:**165 (1964).

52.   Smith, B. T., Torday, J. S. and Giroud, C. J. P. *Steroids* **22:**515 (1973).

53.   Thrash, C. R. and Cunningham, D. D. *Nature* **242:**399 (1973).

54.   Armelin, H. *Proc. Nat. Acad. Sci.* **70:**2702 (1973).

55.   Gospodarowicz, D. *Nature* **249:**123 (1974).

56.   Bresciani, F. *Cell Tissue Kinet.* **1:**51 (1968).

ACKNOWLEDGMENTS

The expert technical assistance of Barbara Sharf and Joan Kabakjian in various parts of these studies is gratefully acknowledged.

2

Placenta as an Aging Organ

PEDRO ROSSO, M.D.

Institute of Human Nutrition, College of Physicians and Surgeons, Columbia University, New York, New York

Many current theories imply an altered RNA metabolism and altered protein metabolism as the basic mechanism of aging (1-7). However, the specific changes that occur in RNA and protein synthesis during aging are still largely undefined. Further, available results show so many discrepancies that one cannot draw any general conclusions. To some extent this state of the art reflects the lack of adequate models for the study of aging.

Current knowledge of the characteristics and mechanisms of aging stems from two main sources: studies done in animals and studies done in tissue culture. In the animal models certain characteristics of aging animals are compared to those of younger animals. Interpreting these data is complicated by the difficulty of isolating changes due to aging per se from changes secondary to aging in other tissues or systems, such as hormonal or vascular changes. Although the influences of vascular changes or hormones are not present in a tissue culture, such a system presents problems even more basic and complex than those in the animal models. In tissue culture the investigator must define the onset of aging, the phenomenon whose unknown characteristics are being explored. At present the basis for defining this onset is debatable.

The study of the interaction between nutrition and aging implies additional problems of experimental design. In tissue culture the problem is to malnourish cells maintained in artificial media in a way that is relevant to an *in vivo* situation. In animal models the problem is again to isolate the direct effect of aging and nutrition in one tissue from possible secondary effects due to interaction of these two factors in other organs or systems. Some of these difficulties could be solved if the interaction of nutrition and aging were studied in an organ that, ideally, shows well-defined temporal changes in function, is readily accessible, is susceptible to experimental manipulation both *in vitro* and *in vivo,* and consists of a uniform population of cells (8). The placenta meets all but the last of these requirements, and it offers in addition the unique advantage of being an organ that grows and apparently ages inside the mature nongrowing and nonaging organism. In spite of these characteristics and the fact that the use of placenta as a model for aging was first discussed two decades ago (9-11), the placenta has not yet been used as a model of an aging organ. In this chapter, normal placental growth and the changes that characterize placental aging will be analyzed and compared with changes found in placenta during maternal malnutrition. It is hoped that this analysis will shed some light on the mechanisms by which aging and malnutrition may interact at an organ level.

PLACENTAL GROWTH AND DEVELOPMENT

Placental growth follows the same sequence described for other organs: first a phase of cell division or a hyperplastic phase, followed by a hypertrophic phase of growth in which cells are enlarging their cytoplasmic mass. Linking these two phases is a transition period in which the end of the hyperplastic phase and the beginning of the hypertrophic phase overlap (12).

In rat placenta the hyperplastic phase of growth lasts 17 days of a total gestation period of 21 days (13), whereas in humans it lasts approximately 36 weeks of a total period of gestation of 40 weeks (14). This sequence of events was demonstrated using total DNA content of the placenta as an index of cell number and protein/DNA ratios or weight/DNA ratios as an index of "cell size." In rat placenta DNA content increases until day 17 of gestation and remains constant thereafter. Thymidine uptake (13), autoradiographic studies (15), and studies of the levels of placental DNA polymerase activity (16) have demonstrated that the leveling off of the DNA curve represents cessation of DNA synthesis and not a steady state of cell loss and renewal.

The RNA and protein content of rat placenta continues to increase after DNA synthesis has stopped at day 17 of gestation, indicating that the placenta is undergoing its hypertrophic phase of growth. The content of both substances continues to increase until day 21 of pregnancy (13). In spite of the continuous increment in RNA and protein content, the rate of synthesis of these two products decreases with age. There are no data available from rat placenta on this phenomenon, but *in vitro* studies of human placenta have demonstrated a progressive decline, with advancing gestational age, in the rate of synthesis of both RNA and protein (17).

The concentration of polyamines also decreases in rat placenta with advancing gestational age (18). The cellular role of polyamines is not well understood although the concentration of these substances in several tissues is higher during periods of rapid RNA synthesis (19). Therefore, the reported decline in polyamine concentration may be reflecting a reduced rate of RNA synthesis.

The progressive reduction in the rate of RNA and protein synthesis and in the concentration of polyamines seems to be part of a more general phenomenon of progressive reduction in the over-all metabolic rate of the placenta. This is best reflected by a progressive reduction of the rate of oxygen consumption *in vitro* reported for both human and rat placenta (20, 21) (Fig. 1). In addition in human placenta the rate of glucose utilization, the rate of production and utilization of pyruvate, the production of lactate, and glycogen concentration also decrease with advancing gestational age (10).

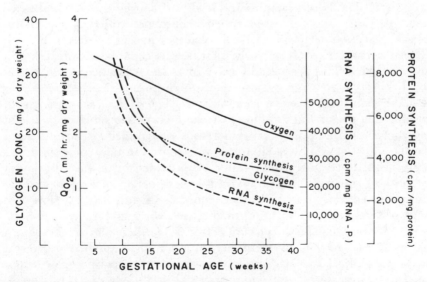

Figure 1. Changes in oxygen consumption (10), glycogen content (10), and rate of RNA and protein synthesis (17) in human placenta during normal gestation.

PLACENTAL FUNCTION DURING NORMAL PREGNANCY

Based on our current knowledge of human placenta, placental function can be divided into two main categories: endocrine functions and transfer functions. The endocrine functions seem to be responsible for most of the adaptive mechanisms found in the maternal organisms during pregnancy; therefore endocrine function influences the fetus mainly indirectly and is mediated by maternal changes. By contrast, the transfer functions are directly responsible for fetal growth. There are few reports on the rate of transfer of substances at different gestational ages. It has been shown in the rat and several other mammalian species, including man, that the permeability of placenta to sodium increases considerably up to nine-tenths of the total period of gestation but falls off between that time and term (22, 23). One known exception to this pattern is the sow, where transfer of sodium into the fetus continues to increase until term (22). Another substance whose transfer characteristics during gestation have been reported is urea; in the sheep urea transfer continues to increase until term (24).

Placental transfer of certain nutrients such as glucose and amino acids during gestation has been studied only in the rat. The transfer of α-aminoisobutyric acid (AIB), a nonmetabolizable amino acid, and glucose, expressed as number of molecules crossing into the fetus per gram of placenta, increases approximately one-hundredfold between day 14 and day 20 of gestation and levels off between day 20 and day 21 of gestation (25). This increased transfer does not reflect solely an increased placental permeability but probably a process of maturation in which the placenta progressively increases its capacity to transfer glucose and AIB. This is especially valid for AIB. It has been demonstrated that AIB is transported into the human placenta and other tissues by energy-consuming active mechanisms (26, 27). Therefore, it is conceivable that the amount of energy consumed in transporting AIB and in general all the amino acids increases in parallel to the increased transfer (Fig. 2). There is an apparent paradox in this, since the extra energy consumed in transport must be provided by a placenta that at the peak of transport function is at its lowest metabolic level. Parallel to the increased rate of transfer between day 14 and day 21 there is a spurt of fetal growth with an approximately thirtyfold increase in body weight. These changes in placental transfer and fetal growth suggest that in the rat the conceptus undergoes a bimodal sequence of growth. In the first phase the placenta is engaged in hyperplastic growth and concentrates most of its metabolic activity in cell division. In this phase transfer of nutrients into the fetus per gram of placental tissue is at a

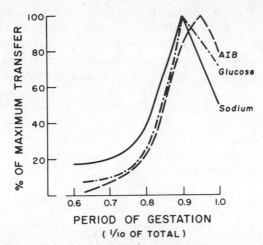

Figure 2. Changes in the rate of transfer of AIB, glucose, and sodium (25, 22) across the rat placenta per gram of placental tissue during normal gestation.

minimum level, although, of course, it is still adequate to maintain normal fetal growth. In the second phase, which coincides with the hypertrophic phase of placental growth, the placenta fully develops its capacity to transfer nutrients and fetal body weight begins to increase rapidly, accelerated by a sudden flow of nutrients.

Another finding, a reduced concentration of tritium and AIB in fetal tissues at day 21 compared with day 20 of gestation (25), suggests that near term the placental capacity to transfer nutrients into the fetus may reach a critical level. This may be due to either a leveling off of the functional capacity of the placenta which, therefore, is unable to meet the increasing requirements of the fetus, or the beginning of a functional decline of the organ. Data that will be discussed in the next sections demonstrate that there is in fact a reduction in the capacity of the placenta to transfer nutrients near term. Therefore, from the point of view of the transfer functions, placental aging begins near term when, paradoxically, absolute requirements of the fetus are the highest.

The endocrine functions of the placenta are measured by the rate of urinary excretion of the different hormones or their plasma levels during pregnancy. Most of our current information derives from human studies. The output of nonprotein hormones, such as progesterone (28, 29) and the estrogens (30), increases constantly until term. In contrast, the levels of protein hormones, such as human chorionic gonadotropins (HCG) and human chorionic somatomammotropin (HCS), have a tendency to decline toward term (31, 32). Thus, the reduction in placental metabolism and transfer functions during late pregnancy is paralleled only by a decline in the excretion of HCG and HCS but not in the excretion of the nonprotein hormones (Fig. 3).

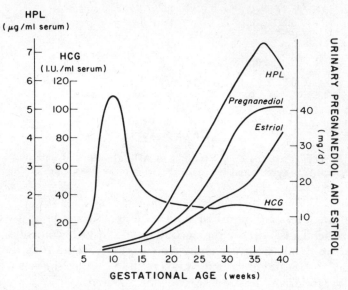

Figure 3. Secretion of some nonprotein and protein hormones by human placenta during the course of gestation (29, 30, 31, 32).

The data on placental transfer and hormone secretion during pregnancy suggest that placental aging is a selective process where certain functions are preserved, or even increased, while others decline.

FUNCTIONAL ASPECTS OF PLACENTAL AGING

The main function of the placenta as an organ is to maintain normal fetal growth. Therefore, the measurement of fetal growth would seem to be a useful way to assess placental function. Unfortunately, the wide range of normal variation of fetal growth as reflected in birth weight prevents the routine use of birth weight as a clinical tool to assess placental function, except in extreme cases of fetal growth retardation.

In several species, including man, it has been observed that the curve of prenatal increments in body weight falls off near term and recovers again postnatally (33, 34). So far the pig is the only known exception to this phenomenon (33). The falling off of the weight curve suggests that the capacity of the placenta to maintain optimal fetal growth is declining near term (Fig. 4). In many cases when gestation continues beyond normal limits spontaneously in man, or in hormonally induced prolonged gestation in the rat and in the rabbit, the fetuses are growth-retarded compared with the postnatal growth of offspring delivered at term and show signs of nutrient deficiency (35–37). Thus, the mechanisms that are causing the slight fall off of the weight curve near term continue to operate after term with a considerable growth-retarding effect on the fetus. During progesterone-induced prolonged gestation in the rat, transfer of AIB and glucose from the maternal circulation into the fetus has been found to be markedly reduced (38). The reduction in the rate of transfer was first noticeable at day 21, and became more evident at day 22 of gestation (Fig. 5). The functional decline in the transfer of AIB and glucose into the fetus begins late in gestation and continues its course during prolonged gestation. The role of the placenta in this decline of transfer has not been completely elucidated. Besides a reduced functional capacity of the placenta, it is conceivable that a reduced rate of placental blood perfusion with increasing gestational age may cause a similar drop in the rate of trans-

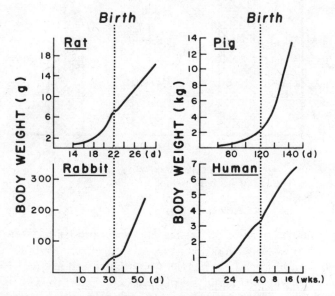

Figure 4. Prenatal and postnatal body weight of the fetuses and offspring in rat (unpublished observations), pig (33), rabbit (34), and man (33).

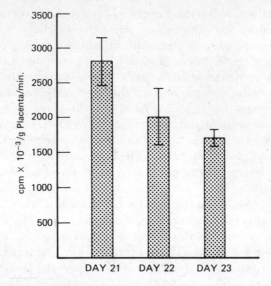

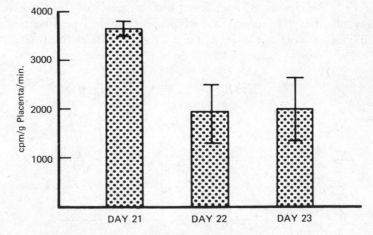

Figure 5. Rate of transfer of glucose (*A*) and AIB (*B*) across the placenta near term and during progesterone-induced prolonged gestation in the rat (38).

fer. Unfortunately, because of its size and the number of fetuses, it is impossible using available methods to get an accurate estimate of placental circulation in the rat. It has been demonstrated in the sheep that the amount of blood perfusing the placenta continues to increase until term (39). The hemodynamic changes in the uterine circulation found in the sheep are remarkably similar to those described in the goat.

Therefore, it is likely that in other species besides the sheep, placental blood perfusion also continues to increase until term. However the higher ratio of placental to fetal concentration of AIB at days 22 and 23 than at day 21 suggests that in the rat reduced placental capacity to transfer AIB and glucose is responsible for the reduced transfer of these substances during prolonged gestation (Fig. 6). This higher ratio indicates that the release of AIB from the placenta into the fetal circulation is delayed during prolonged gestation.

During spontaneously occurring prolonged gestation in humans the plasma concentration of the main placental hormones remains at term levels except for HCS, whose levels are significantly reduced (40). Thus during prolonged gestation most of the endocrine functions do not seem to be as affected as the transfer functions.

METABOLIC ASPECTS OF PLACENTAL AGING

During hormonally induced prolonged gestation in the rat placental DNA content remains at the same level as at day 20 of gestation, indicating that there is no reduction in cell number during placental aging (41). A similar finding has been reported in the brain of the aging mouse (42). Cytoplasmic mass in rat placenta remains constant, as indicated by a constant content of proteins between day 21 and day 23 of gestation (41). These phenomena indicate that any decline in the

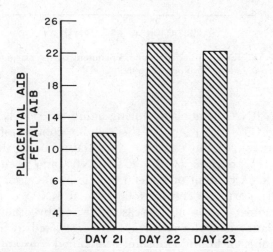

Figure 6. Placental/fetal ratio of AIB concentrations near term and during progester-one-induced prolonged gestation in the rat (38).

metabolic activity of the organ reflects reduced efficiency of the cells and not reduced cytoplasmic mass. In contrast RNA content of each cell decreases markedly (41) (Fig. 7). Since in most tissues ribosomal RNA represents more than 60% of total RNA, the reduced RNA content probably reflects a reduced ribosomal RNA content although it is likely that other types of RNA are also reduced.

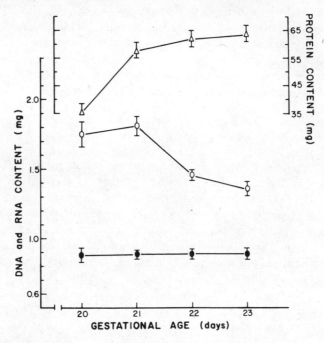

Figure 7. DNA (●), RNA (○) and protein (Δ) content of rat placenta near term and during progesterone-induced prolonged gestation (41).

Changes in RNA metabolism during aging are poorly documented. In the aging C57 BL/6J mouse the cellular content of RNA of the brain remains remarkably constant, the striatum being the only region in which a 10% decline of the RNA/DNA ratio occurred (43). In contrast the RNA content of skeletal muscle in the aging rat decreases markedly (44). In tissue culture total cellular RNA content has been reported by some authors to increase (45) and by others to decrease (46). In the latter case the reduction was restricted to free ribosomes while the number of bound ribosomes remained constant. Research on the rate of synthesis and reproduction of RNA during aging has shown that in the aged mouse there is an increased rate of incorporation of labeled cytidine into both nuclear and cytoplasmic RNA in heart, liver, and kidney (47). However, with longer periods of labeling it has been found that there is no difference between young and aged animals (48). Further, the rate of degradation of ribosomal RNA was found to be similar in young and aged animals in a variety of tissues (48). The higher incorporation with short periods of labeling can be caused by differences in pool size determined by age, but it may also reflect a faster rate of turnover of certain species of RNA. This possibility will be discussed further in the next sections.

The mechanisms by which the concentration of RNA is reduced in the placental tissue during prolonged gestation have not been explored yet. However, it has been found that with increasing gestational age there is a progressive elevation of alkaline ribonuclease activity (RNase) in placenta (41). The role of this enzyme *in vivo* is still undefined. It has been proposed that together with a specific inhibitor it may have a regulatory role for cellular content of RNA (49). This hypothesis remains unproven in spite of the fact that in many situations in which RNA catabolism is increased, alkaline RNase activity is elevated, and vice versa. For example, during development RNase activity in rat liver decreases while cellular content of RNA increases (50). A similar inverse correlation between RNA content and RNase activity has been described in human placenta (51) and rat placenta (52). In rat placenta the increments in the levels of RNase with prolonged gestation coincide with the progressive reduction in the cellular concentration of RNA (Fig. 8).

If RNA metabolism is altered it is likely that protein metabolism will also be altered. In spite of the fact that some of the most popular theories envision aging as a progressive alteration beginning at the level of DNA synthesis and subsequently compromising RNA metabolism and finally protein synthesis, the available data on the changes in protein metabolism during aging are scanty and inconclusive. For example, it has been found that the *in vivo* rate of protein synthesis as measured by the incorporation of ^{3}H-leucine into protein, is higher in livers of 23- to 28-month-old rats than in livers of 11- to 14-month-old rats (53). In contrast, *in vivo* incorporation of leucine into rat skeletal muscle decreases considerably with age (54). Further, the decreased incorporation of leucine into protein seems to reflect not only a loss of ribosomes, but also a reduced ability of the ribosomes to promote synthesis (55, 56). However, these results should be cautiously interpreted since measurement of protein synthesis *in vitro* presents certain difficulties, for example, the possibility that a higher concentration of alkaline ribonuclease will hydrolize RNA during the incubation period. This has been shown to occur in liver of hypophysectomized rats (57).

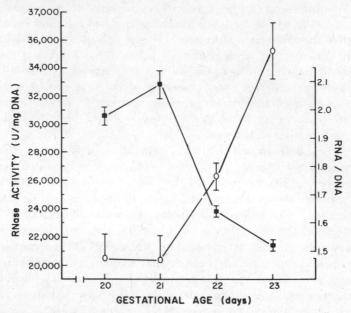

Figure 8. RNase activity (o) and RNA/DNA ratio (■) of rat placenta near term and during prolonged gestation (41).

In rat placenta the rate of protein synthesis, measured *in vivo* by incorporation of ^{14}C-leucine into protein, decreases considerably near term and during prolonged gestation (41).

As we have noted, the concentration of polyamines in placenta, as well as in other tissues, seems to be related to the rate of RNA synthesis or, in general, to the cellular content of RNA. Between day 20 and day 23 of gestation there is a marked reduction of the placental concentration of putrescine and, to a lesser extent, spermidine. In contrast spermine concentration is not affected; hence the spermidine/spermine ratio of the placenta decreases during prolonged gestation (41) (Fig. 9). Such a drop in putrescine concentration during aging has not been reported by others, but the reduction of the spermidine/spermine ratio has been shown in every organ of the rat except brain during normal development up to maturity (58), and more recently also in aging animals (59).

MATERNAL MALNUTRITION AND PLACENTAL METABOLISM

A deficiency of nutrients has been shown to interfere with cell division. As a consequence if a growing animal is undernourished during the hyperplastic phase of growth it will have fewer cells in each of its organs (60). As previously mentioned, the placenta in both the rat and the human is actively engaged in cell division for more than two-thirds of the entire length of pregnancy. Therefore it is as susceptible as any other growing organ to the effects of undernutrition. A reduced placental DNA content has been found in rats fed a low-casein diet throughout pregnancy (61), and also in women from low socioeconomic groups in developing countries who were presumably affected by some degree of undernutrition (62). The reduction in DNA content is a moderate one. This probably explains why in human populations, where normally great individual variation in placental growth is to be expected, no significant changes in the DNA content of placentas from low- and middle-income groups has been reported (63).

In contrast to DNA, RNA metabolism seems to be more susceptible to the effects of maternal malnutrition. In the study in which the placentas from women belonging to two different socioeconomic levels were compared (63), the most significant change reported was a shift in the polysomal profiles to a higher proportion of free ribosomes. The ability to synthesize protein per milligram of RNA in these two groups was similar, suggesting that only the quantity and not the quality of

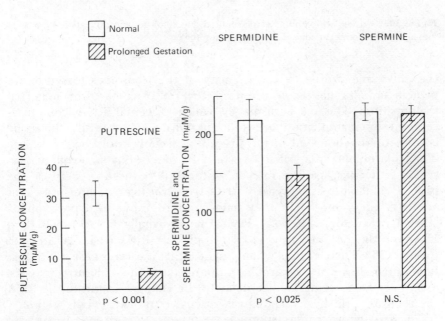

Figure 9. Concentration of putrescine, spermidine, and spermine in rat placenta at day 20 of normal gestation and at day 23 of progesterone-induced prolonged gestation (41).

RNA was affected. In rats fed a low-casein diet there is a clear reduction of the cellular concentration of RNA in the placenta, reflected by a decreased RNA/DNA ratio in this organ (64) (Fig. 10). No analysis of

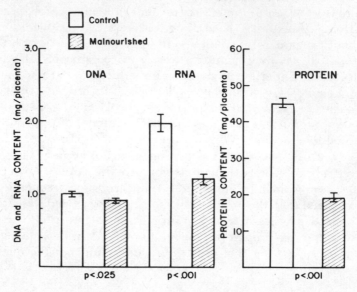

Figure 10. Nucleic acid content of placenta at day 20 of gestation in rats fed a normal diet and a 6% casein diet since day 5 of gestation (64).

the polysomal profile or the capacity of the ribosomes to synthesize protein *in vitro* has been reported for rat placenta after maternal malnutrition. The mechanisms by which placental RNA content is reduced by malnutrition are still unknown. Theoretically the same considerations discussed in the preceding section would be valid here. Thus, placental content of RNA would be reduced by maternal malnutrition either because the rate of synthesis is reduced or because the rate of catabolism is increased. Data from rat liver demonstrate that animals fed a low-casein diet have a more rapid incorporation of labeled precursors into total RNA than normally fed controls (65). However the rate of turnover of cytoplasmic RNA is similar in both groups (66). These results would suggest that a certain type of RNA is being turned over more rapidly in the nuclei of the malnourished rats, a finding that is remarkably similar to the changes found in the RNA metabolism of the liver in aging rats discussed in the previous section.

The activity of alkaline ribonuclease also increases in the placentas of undernourished women (67), but since there is no apparent reduction in the concentration of RNA in these placentas it is difficult to relate ribonuclease activity to RNA concentration in this situation. However, the fact that RNA content is not reduced does not rule out the possibility that RNA catabolism may be increased, although not to the extent of affecting RNA content.

The concentration of polyamines in the malnourished placenta has been measured only in the rat. Similar to the prolonged gestation situation, it has been found that putrescine is markedly reduced without concomitant changes in the concentrations of spermidine and spermine (64). The apparent paradox of this fact, in which a reduction of the amount of precursors does not affect the concentration of products, is still unexplained.

MATERNAL MALNUTRITION AND PLACENTAL FUNCTION

This is a new field in which some results have become available only recently. In rats fed a low-casein diet, since day 5 of gestation, it was found that placental transfer of AIB (68) (Fig. 11) and glucose (64) was markedly reduced when compared to normally fed animals. As in studies done during prolonged gestation it was not known whether blood perfusion to the placenta was affected during maternal malnutrition. However, again an altered placental/fetal concentration ratio of AIB suggests that the placental capacity to release AIB into the fetal circulation is altered.

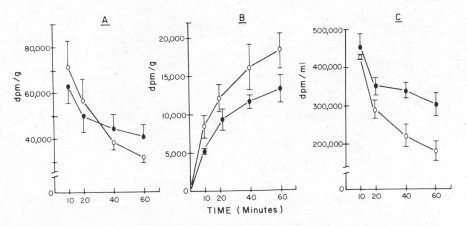

Figure 11. Concentration of AIB in placenta (*A*), fetuses (*B*), and maternal plasma (*C*) in rats fed a normal diet (o) and a 6% casein diet (•) determined by injecting labeled AIB into the maternal circulation at different time intervals (68).

Endocrine functions of the placenta during maternal malnutrition have not been extensively explored. One report, demonstrating reduced urinary excretion of estriol in malnourished mothers, suggests that they may also be altered (69).

CONCLUSIONS

The placenta undergoes a series of metabolic and functional changes during its short life span that mimic the developmental changes that occur in other organs during a much longer period of time. Near term the placenta considerably reduces its capacity to transfer nutrients and its over-all metabolic activity. As a result fetal growth is affected. When gestation is artificially prolonged the transfer function declines further. Parallel to these changes, near term and during prolonged gestation the placenta suffers a reduction in RNA content with a parallel increase in RNase, a reduced rate of protein synthesis, and a reduced concentration of polyamines.

Although most of these changes are similar to changes found in aging tissues it has not been established yet if they in fact reflect the phenomenon of placental aging or if they are only a consequence of a certain degree of normal vascular insufficiency occurring near term.

Table 1   Effects of Aging and Malnutrition on Some Biochemical and Functional Parameters of the Rat Placenta[a]

	Aging	Malnutrition
Biochemical Changes		
DNA content	0	–
RNA content	–	–
Protein content	–	–
RNase activity	+	+
Polyamine concentration:		
putrescine	–	–
spermidine	–	0
spermine	0	0
Functional Changes		
Glucose transfer	–	–
AIB transfer	–	–

[a] 0 = no changes; – = reduced; + = increased.

Some of the biochemical changes found to occur with prolonged gestation, such as a reduced concentration of cellular RNA and increased levels of alkaline ribonuclease, have also been described in rat placenta after ligation of the uterine artery (70). Thus, it is crucial, before the placenta can be accepted as a model for aging, to know in detail the hemodynamic changes that occur in placental blood perfusion during gestation.

Prolonged gestation and maternal malnutrition result in several changes in the placenta that are remarkably similar. These changes are listed in Table 1. The available data in placenta are still too fragmentary to determine whether malnutrition may potentiate the changes that occur with old age. However, some of the results discussed in this paper, such as those in RNA metabolism, suggest that aging and malnutrition may affect cell function at the same levels. Therefore, it is likely that malnutrition may in fact have a synergistic effect on the changes produced by aging in the placenta.

REFERENCES

1. Orgel, L. E. *Proc. Nat. Acad. Sci.* **49:**517 (1963).
2. Hahn, H. P. von. *Adv. Geront. Res.* **3:**1 (1971).
3. Strehler, B., Hirsch, G., Gusseck, D., Johnson, R., and Bick, M. *J. Theor. Biol.* **33:**429 (1971).
4. Curtis, H. J. *Adv. Genet.* **16:**305 (1971).
5. Walford, R. L. Musksgaard, Copenhagen, (1969).
6. Hart, J. W. and Carpenter, D. *Am. Lab.* **3:**31 (1971).
7. Sacher, G. A. *Exper. Geront.* **3:**265 (1968).
8. Bellamy, D. *Gerontologia* **19:**162 (1973).
9. Huggett, A. St. G., *Ciba Colloquia in Ageing,* Vol. 2, 1956, pp. 118.
10. Villee, C. A., In *Ciba Colloquia in Ageing,* Vol. 2, 1956, pp. 129.
11. Wislocki, G. B. In *Ciba Colloquia in Ageing,* Vol. 2, 1956, pp. 105.
12. Winick, M. and Noble A. *Develop. Biol.* **12:**451 (1965).
13. Winick, M. and Noble, A. *Nature* **212:**5057 (1966).
14. Winick, M., Coscia, A., and Noble, A. *Pediatrics* **39:**248 (1967).
15. Jollie, W. P. *Am. J. Anat.* **114:**161 (1964).
16. Velasco, E. G. and Brasel, J. A. *J. Pediatrics* **86:**274 (1975).
17. Beaconsfield, P., Ginsburg, J., and Jeacock, M. K. *Develop. Med. Child. Neurol.* **6:**469, (1964).
18. Gunaga, K. P., Sheth, A. R., Gunaga, C. K., and Rao, S. S. *Indian J. Biochem. Biophys* **10:**134 (1973).
19. Bachrach, U. In *Function of Naturally Occurring Polyamines* U. Bachrach, Ed. Academic, New York, 1973, p. 74.
20. Wang, H. W. and Hellman L. M. *Bull. Johns Hopk. Hosp.* **73:**31 (1943).

21.   Bde, F. *Acta Obstet. Gynecol. Scand.* **22** Suppl. 2, p. 1 (1942).

22.   Gellhorn, A. and Flexner, L. B. *Am. J. Physiol.* **136:**750 (1942).

23.   Flexner, L. B., Cowie, D. B., Hellman, L. M., Wilde, W. S., and Vosburgh, G. J. *Am. J. Obstet. Gynec.* **55:**469, (1948).

24.   Kuhanek, J. F., Meschia, G., Makowski, E. L., and Battaglia, F. *Am. J. Physiol.* **226:**1257 (1974).

25.   Rosso, P. *Am. J. Obstet. Gynec.* (In press) (1975).

26.   Litonjua, A. D., Caneas, M., Soliman, J., and Paulino, D. Q. *Am. J. Obstet.* **99:**242 (1967).

27.   Christensen, H. N. *Fed. Proc.* **32:**19 (1973).

28.   Eton, B. and Short, R. V. *J. Obstet. Gynec. Brit. Emp.* **67:**785 (1960).

29.   Shearman, R. P. *J. Obstet. Gynec. Brit. Emp.* **66:**1 (1959).

30.   Klopper, A. and Billewicz, W. *J. Obstet. Gynec. Brit. Common.* **70:**1024 (1963).

31.   Mishell, D. R. Jr., Wide, L., and Gemzell, C. A. *J. Clin. Endocr.* **23:**125 (1963).

32.   Garoff, L. and Seppala, M. *J. Obstet. Gynec. Brit. Comm.* **80:**695 (1973).

33.   Widdowson, E. M. In *Biology of Gestation*, vol. 2. N. S. Assali, Ed., Academic, New York, 1968, p. 1.

34.   Dawes, G. S. In *Foetal and Neonatal Physiology*, G. S. Dawes, Ed., Year Book Medical Publishers, Chicago, 1969, p. 42.

35.   Clifford, S. H. *J. Pediat.* **44:**1 (1954).

36.   Bührdel, P., Willgerodt, H., Keller, E., Theile, H., and Emmrich, P. *Biol. Neonate* **24:**57 (1974).

37.   Willgerodt, H., Keller, E., Theile, H., and Beyreiss, K. Wiss, Z. Friedr-Schiller Univ. Jena, Math Naturwiss, R. **21:**701 (1972).

38.   Rosso, P. *Am. J. Obstet. Gynec.* (In press) (1975).

39.   Rosenfeld, C. R., Morriss, F. H. Jr., Makowski, E. L., Meschia, G., and Battaglia, F. *Gynecol. Invest.* **5:**252 (1974).

40.   Hobbins, J. C., Goldstein, L., and Hofchild, J. *Gynecol. Invest.* **5:**49 (1974).

41.   Rosso, P. *Pediat. Res.* **9:**279 (1975).

42.   Franks, L. M., Wilson, P. D., and Whelan, R. D. *Gerontologia* **20:**21 (1974).

43.   Chacones, G. and Finch, C. E. *J. Neurochem* **21:**1469 (1973).

44.   Breuer, C. B. and Florini, J. R. *Biochem.* **4:**1544 (1965).

45.   Cristofalo, V. J. *Adv. Gerontol. Res.* **4:**45 (1972).

46.   Robbins, E., Levine, E. M., and Eagle, H. *J. Exp. Med.* **131:**1211 (1970).

47.   Wulff, V. J., Samis, H. V. Jr., and Falzone, J. A. *Adv. Gerontol. Res.* **2:**37 (1967).

48.   Menzies, R. A., Misha, R. A., and Gold, P. H. *Mech. Aging Dev.* **1:**117 (1972).

49.   Kraft, N. and Shortman, K. *Biochim. Biophys, Acta.* **217:**164 (1970).

50.   Rosso, P., Nelson, M., and Winick, M. *Growth* **37:**143 (1973).

51.   Brody, S. *Biochim. Biophys. Acta* **24:**502 (1957).

52.   Velasco, E. (personal communication).

53.   Beauchene, R. L., Roeder, L. M., and Barrows, C. H. Jr. *J. Gerontol.* **25:**359 (1970).

54.   Srivastava, U. and Chaudhary, K. D. *Can. J. Biochem.* **47:**231 (1969).

55.   Britton, G. W. and Sherman, F. G. *Exper. Geront.* **10:**67 (1975).

56.   Buetow, D. E. and Gandhi, P. S. *Exp. Geront.* **8:**243 (1973).

57. Brewer, E. N., Foster, L. B., and Sells, B. H. *J. Biol. Chem.* **244:**1380 (1969).

58. Jänne, J., Raina, A., and Sümes, N. *Acta Physiol. Scand.* **62:**352 (1964).

59. Ferioli, M. E. and Comolli, R. *Exper. Geront.* **10:**13 (1975).

60. Winick, M. and Noble, M. *J. Nutrition* **89:**300 (1966).

61. Winick, M. In *Diagnosis and Treatment of Fetal Disorders.* K. Adamsons, Ed., Springer-Verlag, N. Y. 1969, p. 83.

62. Dayton, D. H., Filer, L. J., and Canosa, C. *Fed. Proc.* **28:**488 (1966).

63. Laga, E., Driscoll, S., and Munro, H. *Pediatrics* **50:**33 (1972).

64. Rosso, P., Wasserman, M., Rozovoski, J., and Velasco, E. *Clin. Chem.* (In press) (1975).

65. Quirin-Stricker, C. and Mandel, P. *Bull. Soc. Chim. Biol.* **50:**31 (1968).

66. Wanemacher, R. W. Jr., Wannemacher, C. F., and Yatvin, M. B. *Biochem. J.* **124:**385 (1971).

67. Velasco, E., Rosso, P., Brasel, J. A., and Winick, M. *Am. J. Obstet. Gynec.* (In press) (1975).

68. Rosso, P. *Science* **187:**648 (1975).

69. Iyengar, L. *Am. J. Obstet. Gynec.* **102:**834 (1968).

70. Velasco, E. G., Brasel, J. A., Sigulem, D. M., Rosso, P., and Winick, M. *J. Nutr.* **103:**213 (1973).

3

Nutrition and Longevity in Experimental Animals

MORRIS H. ROSS

The Institute for Cancer Research, The Fox Chase Cancer Center, Philadelphia, Pennsylvania

The health-promoting and life-prolonging role of nutrition has attracted attention since ancient times. Some of the consequences of gluttony were recorded even then, as attested to by the homilies extolling the virtues of moderation. Despite the limitations of modern actuarial reports and early experimental findings, the data do show that obesity shortens lifespan and that limitation in food or caloric intake can result in longer life (1-11). The effects of chronic restriction in food intake on laboratory animals have been so apparent that it is difficult to avoid concluding that no environmental factor so decisively reduces the rate or expression of the aging processes. In our laboratory, we have been able to nearly double the life expectancy of male rats by imposing a regimen of severe underfeeding throughout the animal's postweaning life (Fig. 1). In fact some animals survived more than 1800 days; for the human this would correspond to approximately 180 years.

The reduction in frequency and severity of some diseases of age, associated with chronic restriction, is even more striking (5, 7-10, 12-24). Glomerulonephrosis rarely occurs in calorically restricted rats, whereas in full-fed rats this highly debilitating age-dependent kidney disease is found in as many as 40% of the animals (20). Myocardial

This investigation was supported by Public Health Service Research Grant Nos. RR-05539 and CA-06927 from the National Institute of Health and by an appropriation from the Commonwealth of Pennsylvania.

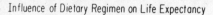

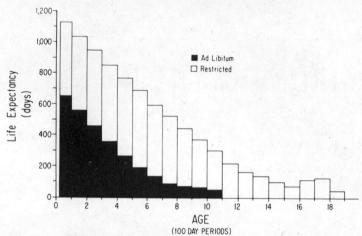

Figure 1.   Life expectancy of male rats fed a purified diet in ad libitum and in restricted amounts throughout postweaning life. Intake of restricted rats limited to approximately 30% of the mean intake of rats fed ad libitum. Number of individually housed Charles River COBS rats: 175 for the ad libitum group and 200 for the restricted group. Composition of the diet: 22% casein, 58.5% sucrose, 13.5% corn oil, 6% salt mixture (USP XII). For vitamin and trace element content see (21).

fibrosis, peribronchial lymphocytosis, periarteritis, prostatitis, and endocrine hyperplasias are among the diseases that are decreased by 50 to 90% and the relatively few cases that do occur are usually mild and develop at very late ages (9, 10, 19). The effect of limiting the amount of food consumed on the incidence of tumors and on the age of the animal when they occur differs depending on tumor type: The processes involved in the development of some tumors are so diet-sensitive that these tumors occur infrequently or not at all (16, 21, 24). However, there are some tumors that are not affected and still others for which the incidence is actually increased (Table 1).

The adverse effects of severe underfeeding cannot be overlooked and are serious enough to militate against recommending this practice for the human. Aside from the fact that a higher proportion of tumors that occur in restricted animals are malignant, there is an increase in infant mortality, stunting of growth and accompanying impairment in structural, functional, and behavioral development, and a greater susceptibility to bacterial and parasitic diseases (25–34).

The observations on laboratory animals are important insofar as they indicate that it is possible to extend the period of life prior to the onset of some of the diseases commonly associated with aging. It is therefore

Table 1 Influence of Restriction of Food Intake on Spontaneous Tumor Frequency in the Rat[a]

	Tumor Frequency[b] (Cases in ad libitum group/cases in restricted group)[c]		
	Decreased	Unaffected	Increased
Epithelial (165/97)	Adenoma, all sites (122/54)	Papilloma of urinary bladder (30/27)	Carcinoma, all sites (9/15)
Lymphoreticular and Hemato- poietic (63/30)	Reticulum cell sarcoma of lung (35/8)		Reticulum cell sarcoma of lymph- oid organs (5/12)
	Thymoma (16/2)		
Musculo- skeletal and Soft (33/22)	Lipoma (8/0)	Fibroma, all sites (11/8)	
		Fibrosarcoma, all sites (10/7)	
Endocrine (121/56)	Anterior pituitary (60/12)	Thyroid (15/17)	Adrenal (4/10)
			Parathyroid (1/7)
	Pancreatic islet cells (40/10)		

[a] Males of the Charles River COBS-SD strain.
[b] Tumors classed by tissue origin, primary site, or type.
[c] Combined data of three groups fed ad libitum and three groups fed on a restricted basis. A total of 727 and 735 rats, respectively, were alive at the time the first tumor was found. Total tumor incidence, 35% and 18% for the ad libitum and restricted groups, respectively. For additional information see (21).

reasonable to ask whether there are dietary regimens that will contribute to a reduced rate of aging but that avoid the adverse consequences associated with disturbances of growth and maturational processes. To this end, a series of new long-term experimental studies with the rat were undertaken. In the first of these, isocaloric diets of varying composition were fed in both ad libitum and restricted amounts. The regimens imposed on the animals were begun at weaning age or at progressively later ages until maturity had been reached. In the course of this chapter we will also describe the results of a study in which the animals were permitted to select their own diets.

When the diets are fed in ad libitum amounts throughout postweaning life, the risk of developing an age-related disease is appreciably modified by the composition of the diet. For the nonneoplastic diseases, for example, a fivefold increase in the proportion of dietary protein leads to a dramatic increase in the incidence of renal, myocardial, and prostatic diseases (Table 2). The effects on the frequency

Table 2   Prevalence of Age-Related Disease of Rats as Influenced by the Level of Dietary Protein[a]

	Protein Content of Diet, %		
	10	22	51
	Cases/100 rats		
Glomerulonephrosis[b]	4	18	39
Myocardial fibrosis[b]	< 1	4	18
Prostatitis	5	10	12

[a]All rats fed ad libitum throughout postweaning life. Number of rats entered into the experiment, 250 per group.
[b]Moderate and severe cases.

and age-adjusted risk of tumors differ with the tumor type. An increase in dietary fat increases the incidence of mammary tumors in mice (35–37). A diet presumed to be adequate in all respects is more conducive to the development of tumors of several endocrine organs, and possibly some endocrine-dependent tumors, than a diet which is marginally low or excessively high in protein content (18, 21). This biphasic relationship is especially pronounced for tumors of the anterior pituitary gland, thyroid, and islets of Langerhans. In contrast, the risk of developing urinary bladder tumors, one of the tumor types that is not influenced by caloric intake, is directly related to the level of dietary protein—a fivefold increase in the protein content of the diet is accompanied by a fourfold increase in relative morbidity. Conversely, the risk of developing tumors of the thymus gland decreases by a factor of 8. In addition, as the ratio of carbohydrate decreases, proportionally more of the tumors are malignant.

Since these diets were also fed in restricted isocaloric amounts, it was possible to distinguish the effects of the composition of the diet from the effects of calories. The protein/carbohydrate ratio of the diet can either enhance the disease-inhibitory effects of limitation in food intake or oppose it. For example, the effect of restriction on the incidence of prostatitis is minimal when the diet is low in protein, but substantial when the diet is high in protein (38). For tumors in general, or the malignant forms in particular, the opposite situation prevails in that the effects of restriction are more pronounced at low protein levels (21). Glomerulonephrosis represents an extreme situation. Restriction in food intake so completely overrides the ad libitum protein effect that this renal condition does not occur even among the longest-lived rats.

Life expectancies of rats consuming diets that contain 10, 22, or 51% protein in restricted amounts are consistently greater than the expectancies of rats consuming the same diets in ad libitum amounts (Table 3). The high-protein diet tends to accentuate the effects of restriction and the low-protein diet minimizes them (21). Each type of feeding practice gives rise to a separate relationship between lifespan and protein/carbohydrate ratio, but a single inverse relationship is obtained only when lifespan is related to the actual intake of carbohydrate (Fig. 2). This continuum suggests that the carbohydrate component may be the determining factor rather than caloric intake per se or the absolute or relative intake of the protein component.

Table 3   Influence of the Level of Dietary Protein on Length of Life[a]

Casein Content of Diet, %	Life Expectancy at 21 Days of Age	
	Ad libitum series	Restricted series
	(days)	
10	540	692
22	585	838
51	614	934

[a]For age-specific mortality rates, relative mortality risk values, and experimental conditions see (21).

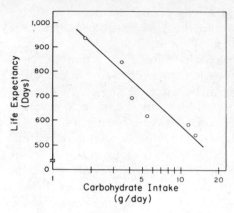

Figure 2. Relationship between life expectancy of male rats and mean daily intake of carbohydrate. A group of 1600 individually housed rats were fed in ad libitum or restricted amounts three complete purified diets differing only in their protein/carbohydrate ratio. The regimens were maintained throughout life beginning at 21 days of age. The composition of the diets and other experimental conditions are described in (18) and (21).

To summarize, it appears that when animals are maintained on a dietary regimen throughout postweaning life, both the quantity and the composition of the diet significantly modify length of life and the susceptibility to diseases of age. However, no two dietary groups, whether fed under ad libitum or under restricted conditions, have the same disease susceptibility even though the caloric intake is identical. Similarly, there is no single regimen that uniformly reduces or increases the frequency of every tumor type; as a consequence, the tumor type spectrum of one dietary population differs from that of another.

The diets and feeding regimens that are compatible with long life when started at time of weaning become progressively less so when begun at later ages (17, 39). A similar phenomenon has been shown for mammary tumors in mice; restriction in intake begun early in life decreases the incidence to a greater extent than when the regimen is begun later in life (40, 41). When dietary intervention is delayed until after rats reach maturity, nearly all diets tested shorten the span of life of the animals (17, 19). Limiting the intake of these diets in varying degrees only accentuates the life-shortening effects. This change in response may represent an age-dependent loss in the ability of the animal to adapt to a new dietary regimen. With one important exception, it would also seem that if a diet is to have a life-prolonging and disease-inhibiting or delaying influence, it will do so only if the diet is begun early in life. This interpretation is supported by the results of a study in which the ad libitum–restriction feeding pattern was reversed. Rats were underfed for the first 7 weeks postweaning, and at 70 days of age they were rehabilitated by permitting them to feed ad libitum for the remainder of their lifetimes. The age-specific mortality rates for these rats are consistently lower than the mortality rates of rats fed the same diet in ad libitum amounts throughout life starting at 21 days of age (24). The over-all improvement in mortality risk attributable to the early period of underfeeding is 20%.

The effects of early underfeeding on the frequency of some diseases of age, particularly tumors, are more impressive. For example, the age-adjusted morbidity of anterior pituitary gland tumors is reduced in the restricted–ad libitum rats by approximately 70% (Table 4) when compared to the risk in rats whose intake was not limited at any age (24). Of the total reduction in incidence of these tumors associated with lifetime underfeeding, the greater part can be ascribed to the effect of restriction during the first 5 to 10% period of the animal's lifetime. Other than reticular cell sarcomas, for which the incidence is slightly increased, the long-lasting effects of early underfeeding are evident in varying degrees for other tumors and diseases common to the strain of rats used.

We could conclude from these observations that the mechanisms through which nutrition influences the aging processes are already operative during the youthful stage of life. The nature of the mechanism is unknown but it may be another expression of the long-lasting effects of early nutrition that have been shown for a variety of developmental processes.

The fact that there is one exception to the rule that a change in diet combined with restriction in intake instituted at mid-life shortens life rather than lengthens it indicated to us that the life-shortening effects

Table 4   Effect of Change in Dietary Regimen on Frequency of Pituitary Adenoma[a]

Dietary Regimen	Number of rats	Chromophobe Adenomas	
		Number of cases	Relative morbidity
D_{22} ad libitum for life	250	26	100
D_{22} restricted for life	250	3	< 1
D_{22} restricted 21-70 days, then ad libitum for life	150	6	28

[a]Experimental conditions and additional actuarial data given in (24).

of a full-feeding regimen during the first half of life can to some extent be overcome. The conditions for modifying lifespan beneficially appear to be highly critical and age-dependent (39). Rats at mid-life provided a diet with a protein/calorie ratio of 1:5 under moderate conditions of restriction have a life expectancy that is almost equivalent to that of rats whose regimen of restriction, instituted at 70 days of age, was considerably more severe. Increasing or decreasing the degree of restriction or modifications in the protein content of the diet shortens rather than lengthens the animal's span of life (17).

Under natural conditions for man and animals, the quantity and composition of the diet consumed normally changes with age. If data from long-term experiments with laboratory animals are to provide guidelines for feeding under nonlaboratory conditions, we must identify the progression of changes in nutritional status throughout life which in toto contributes to a long life relatively free of debilitating diseases of age. The long-lasting effects of early nutritional experiences add to the difficulties of the problem.

A new approach was suggested by the fact that young rats (and several other species) when allowed to choose their own diets do select essential dietary substances in such amounts as to sustain life, to grow, and even to reproduce (42). To the extent that a variety of genetic or induced abberations in the regulation of metabolism early in life are associated with compensatory changes in dietary preference (43–50), the dietary selections appear to be a form of tropism. If the dietary choices and the changes in preference with age do in fact reflect the metabolic requirements of the animal so as to be "conducive to the maintenance of a normal physiological equilibrium" (47), it may be possible to assess the long-term consequences of dietary habits at different stages of life. Moreover, by eliminating the artificially and arbitrarily imposed fixed dietary regimens, this method of feeding more closely simulates the natural condition.

The dietary variables in this experiment were limited to the absolute and relative intake of protein and carbohydrate and to total calories. Instead of being given each of the dietary constituents separately, the individually housed rats were given three complete isocaloric diets in three separate containers. These differed only in their protein and carbohydrate content (21). The amounts consumed from each were determined daily for all rats. Other rats with the same preweaning dietary history maintained under identical environmental conditions were fed in the conventional manner; each rat received only one of the three basal diets throughout life.

Rats permitted to select their own diets consume some food from each of the containers but the absolute and relative amounts taken differ from rat to rat. Most rats establish within the first several weeks the quantity and composition of the diet that they continue to consume over a prolonged period of time. Some require a longer period before they too stabilize their pattern of intake, while still others slowly but continuously change their preferences for protein and carbohydrate. As a result there is a complex spectrum of dietary preferences in which no two of the genetically heterogeneous rats have the same intake pattern, quantitatively or qualitatively (38–51). The rats, however, grow more rapidly, attain higher mature body weights, and have a greater gross efficiency of food utilization than rats fed any one of the fixed diets.

In assessing the mortality data, the actuarial methods of analysis applicable to groups of animals maintained under constant dietary conditions were supplanted by appropriate statistical procedures that permitted the use of ungrouped data. The derivation of simple, partial, and multiple correlation coefficients and regressions allows us to isolate the nature of a relationship between two or more dietary variables while other variables are held statistically constant.

Thus, a highly significant inverse correlation exists between the quantity of food consumed and the duration of life which varies in this group of rats from approximately 300 to 1100 days (Fig. 3) (51). The association is limited to the period encompassing the first half of life. After the animals are fully mature, the amount of food they consume no longer relates inversely to lifespan. The relationship was first detected when the animals had been on the self-selection regimen for only 5 weeks. The "intake effect" is maximal during the 100- to 200-day period (Fig. 4); a 10% difference in daily intake is associated with

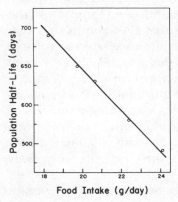

Food Intake (g/day)

Figure 3. Example of the relationship between quantity of food consumed by male rats given freedom of dietary choice and length of life. For the actuarial analysis, rats were classed according to their mean daily intake of food (during the 100 to 199 day age period) irrespectively of the composition of the diet each selected. Population half-life estimated from percent survival curves. For statistical analyses, ungrouped data were used: Correlation coefficient for the association between length of life and food intake at this age period, $r = 0.40$, $p = 0.000005$; regression equation, length of life in days $= 1180 - 26 \times$ mean daily food intake in grams. For experimental conditions, see (51).

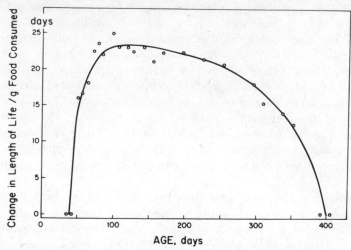

Figure 4. Age limitation when the amount of food consumed by rats given freedom of dietary choice correlates significantly with length of life. At each age period the value shown represents the slope of the best-fit line for the inverse relationship between length of life and mean daily intake of food. Significant correlations obtained only between 50 and 350 days postpartum.

approximately an 8% loss in the probable lifespan. (In terms of the human a difference in the daily intake of 100 to 125 calories during the period of growth would be expected to decrease the duration of life by approximately 2½ years.)

Since the growth of animals depends to a large extent upon the amount of food consumed when the essential components in the diet are present at adequate levels, the relationship between lifespan and body weight should be similar to that for food intake. Body weight early in life proved to be an even more sensitive indicator than food intake. Our data clearly show once more that dietary practices that promote rapidity of growth and early maturation are not conducive to long life. Conversely, for each additional day an animal requires to reach a preassigned weight during the early growth phase, there is a high probability that the future lifespan of the animal will increase by 1⅔ days. When the rats are 15 weeks old, there is an almost one-to-one inverse relationship between body weight and length of life, that is, a 1-gram difference in body weight is associated with a 0.9-day difference in lifespan. Beyond 20 weeks of age, a similar difference in body weight is associated with an appreciably smaller effect on lifespan. After mid-life has been passed, body weight no longer has any significant relationship to the subsequent span of life.

The food intake effect is strengthened or even eliminated depending on the composition of the diet the animal selects. The absolute and relative intakes of protein and carbohydrate relate to length of life independently of one another and not necessarily at the same stage of life (51). Prior to 50 days of age, the protein content of the diet correlates directly with lifespan. It is not until after the animals are 300 to 400 days old that the protein/carbohydrate ratio of the diet again relates to lifespan; however, at this phase of life the association is an inverse one. During the interim period, it is the absolute levels of intake of protein and of carbohydrate that correlate with lifespan. Initially, the two dietary components have nearly equivalent effects. With increasing age, the life-shortening influence of high carbohydrate intake diminishes more rapidly than it does for protein. Beyond 300 days the amount of carbohydrate an animal consumes no longer correlates with lifespan whereas the level of protein intake continues to be a significant factor well into maturity. The life-shortening effect of excessive intake of protein at late ages, however, appears to be of a lower order than it was during the early adult period of life.

The nature of the dietary practices associated with long life may be deduced from the data obtained for discrete age periods. However, we chose to use the retrospective method of analysis to determine the sequential age-related changes in appetite associated with long life and with short life. Two subgroups were formed from the entire group of self-selection rats. In the long-lived subgroup all rats lived at least 714 days, and in the short-lived subgroup no rat lived longer than 550 days. As anticipated, the dietary preferences of the short- and long-lived rats differ quantitatively and qualitatively. The quantity of food consumed by rats in these two classes is similar over the first 4 weeks only. Beyond this age, the mean daily intake of the shortest-lived rats is at least 10% greater than the amount of food taken by rats whose life expectancy is nearly twice as long (mean life spans: 473 and 787 days, respectively).

Qualitatively, the short-lived rats exhibit a progression of changes in preference. The first indication that these animals will have a short lifespan becomes evident by the third week of feeding in that they select diets that are significantly lower in protein content than those chosen by the long-lived rats (51). A change in the protein appetite of these animals occurs when they are approximately 10 weeks old, at which time they tend to prefer diets of higher protein content. By the time the animals are adults they select diets that are even higher in protein content than those chosen by the long-lived rats. In contrast, the protein/carbohydrate ratio of the diets selected by the long-lived animals remains uncommonly constant throughout much of their life-times. If there is any change in preference from one age period to another it is limited to a subtle but statistically nonsignificant decrease in the protein/carbohydrate ratio of the diet selected after the animal reaches the adult stage of life.

These observations point up the potential danger in extending conclusions based on the results with single fixed diets to man or even to rats living under natural conditions. However, these observations do have direct bearing on the interpretation of data obtained with fixed dietary regimens. A single diet may meet the needs of an animal at one age but not at another. A single diet may meet the unique requirements of some, but not all the animals in a dietary group. For the former, the diet imposed may have little effect on what is presumed to be the animal's genetically determined span of life. For those rats whose requirements differ, the same diet may well be beneficial for some and detrimental for others.

From a pragmatic point of view, the immediate question this premise raises is whether dietary intervention applied to the short-lived animals will contribute to a lengthening of their lifespans. Manipulating their diet so as to conform with the dietary selections made by the long-lived rats may, on the other hand, represent for these short-lived rats a state of protein overnutrition early in life and protein undernutrition later in life. If this is not the case, will an increase in protein content of the diet early in life be sufficient, or must the change in regimen involve the later period of life as well? Since with fixed diets increasing levels of dietary protein are associated with an increase in frequency of many of the nonneoplastic diseases and of some tumors, we might ask whether any further advantage would accrue to the long-lived rats if the protein content of their diets was reduced after they reached the adult period of life.

Aside from the fact that the dietary practices of an individual animal correspond closely with its duration of life, the diet each animal chooses has also a "near-determinant" influence on the frequency of some diseases of age that it develops. The rats permitted freedom of choice are considerably more prone to develop tumors and renal, myocardial, and prostatic diseases than rats fed any one of the fixed diets in the conventional manner (38). The self-selection rats are, however, less subject to peribronchial lymphocytosis (Table 5). For some tumors, the incidence is as high as or higher than that found for all three fixed dietary groups combined. There are also some tumor types that we had not previously encountered in animals fed fixed diets. Another surprising facet of this phenomenon is that it does not matter if the animals consume small, moderate, or large amounts of food, or if the diets they select are low, intermediate, or high in protein content; the frequencies are consistently high. It is as if the quantity

Table 5   Prevalence of Age-Related Diseases as Influenced by Mode of Feeding

| | Dietary Regimen[a] | | | |
| | Self-selection | Single - Fixed | | |
	(D_{10}, D_{22}, D_{51})	D_{10}	D_{22}	D_{51}
	Incidence, %			
Tumors, all types	91	29	38	39
Glomerulone-phrosis[b]	56	4	18	39
Myocardial fibrosis[b]	38	< 1	4	18
Prostatitis	62	5	10	12
Peribronchial lymphocytosis	12	34	35	37

[a]Diets identified by the proportion of the protein component in the diet.
[b]Moderate and severe cases only.

and composition of the diet selected by each animal vary in a way that tends to optimize the risk to the individual of developing one or more diseases of age. To paraphrase an old proverb, one man's meat may also be his poison.

The concept of individual specificity in dietary conditions that promote those processes that culminate in age-related diseases implies that individuals whose particular dietary "needs" are critically met are more likely to develop a disease of age than individuals with other needs fed the same diet. If valid, it would follow that to reduce the risk of developing a diet-sensitive disease of late life, the diet must be not only physiologically adequate but "tailored" to the individual instead of the population; that is, if we know the dietary conditions that increase the probability that an individual will develop a disease of age, can we use this information to indicate the type of dietary modifications that should be introduced early in life to reduce the likelihood that the individual will develop such diseases?

Such studies, which also include the genetic aspects of the problem, are in progress, and this approach may resolve to some extent the dichotomy between the nutritionally retarded maturational changes and the life-prolonging and health-promoting effects later in life.

ACKNOWLEDGMENTS

I wish to acknowledge the contributions to this work by my colleague, Dr. Gerrit Bras, of the Faculty of Medicine, University of Utrecht, Netherlands, and of Lucile Sweeny and Mary Cahalan for their technical assistance. Thanks are also due to Hoffman-LaRoche, Inc., Lederle Laboratories, Merck and Company, and Mead Johnson and Company for their generous supply of corn oil and vitamins used in these studies.

REFERENCES

1. Armstrong, D. B., Dublin, I., Wheatley, M., and Marks, H. *J.A.M.A.* **147:**1007 (1951).
2. Katz, L. N., Stamler, J., and Pick, R. *Fed. Proc.* **15:**885 (1956).
3. Build and Blood Pressure Study, Vol. 1. Published by Soc. of Actuaries, Chicago, 1959.
4. Waxler, S. H., Tabar, P., and Melcher, L. *Cancer Res.* **13:**276 (1953).
5. Silberberg, M. and Silberberg, R. *Physiol. Rev.* **35:**347 (1955).
6   Lane, P. W. and Dickie, M. M. *J. Nutr.* **64:**549 (1958).
7. McCay, C. M. In *Cowdry's Problems of Ageing.* A. I. Lansing, Ed., Williams and Wilkins, Baltimore, 1952, p. 139.
8. Carlson, A. J. and Hoelzel, F. *J. Nutr.* **34:**81 (1947).
9. Ross, M. H. *Fed. Proc.* **18:**1190 (1959).
10. Berg, B. N. and Simms, H. S. *J. Nutr.* **71:**255 (1960).
11. Ross, M. H. *J. Nutr.* **7:**197 (1961).
12. Slonaker, J. R. *Am. J. Physiol.* **98:**266 (1931).
13. Saxton, J. A., Jr. and Kimball, G. C. *Arch. Path.* **32:**951 (1941).
14. Rusch, H. P., Kline, B. E. and Bauman, C. A. *Cancer Res.* **5:**431 (1945).
15. Tannenbaum, A. and Silverstone, H. In *Advances in Cancer Research,* Vol. 1. J. P. Greenstein and A. Haddow, Eds., Academic, New York, 1953, p. 451.
16. Ross, M. H. and Bras, G. *J. Nutr.* **87:**245 (1965).
17. Ross, M. H. *Proc. 7th Internat. Congr. Nutr. 1966,* Verlag. Fiedr., Braunschweig, West Germany, p. 35.
18. Ross, M. H., Bras, G., and Ragbeer, M. S. *J. Nutr.* **100:**177 (1970).
19. Ross, M. H. In *Diet and Bodily Constitution.* G. Wolstenholme, Ed., Ciba Foundation Study Group #17. Little Brown, Boston, 1964.
20. Bras, G. and Ross, M. H. *Toxicol. Appl. Pharmacol.* **6:**247 (1964).
21. Ross, M. H. and Bras, G. *J. Nutr.* **103:**944 (1973).
22. Bras, G. and Ross, M. H. *Proc. 7th Internat. Congr. Nutr. 1966,* Verlag. Fiedr., Braunschweig, West Germany, p. 226.
23. White, F. R. *Cancer Res.* **21:**281 (1961).
24. Ross, M. H. and Bras, G. *J. Nat. Cancer Inst.* **47:**1095 (1971).

25. Lat, J., Widdowson, E. M., and McCance, R. A. *Proc. Roy. Soc.*. (Biol.) **153**:347 (1960).

26. Dobbing, J. In *Development of Metabolism as Related to Nutrition*. P. Hahn and O. Koldovsky, Eds., S. Krager, New York, 1960, p. 132.

27. Winick, M. and Coombs, J. In *Ann. Rev. of Medicine*, Vol. 23, 1972, p. 149.

28. Knittle, J. L. and Hirsch, J. *J. Clin. Invest.* **47**:2091 (1968).

29. Heard, C. R. L. and Stewart, R. J. C. *Hormones* **2**:40 (1971).

30. Smythe, P. M. et al. *Lancet* **2**:939 (1971).

31. Novakova, V. et al. *Nature* (London) **193**:280 (1962).

32. Dubos, R., Lee, C. J., and Costello, R. *J. Exp. Med.* **130**:963 (1969).

33. Culley, W. J. and Lineberger, R. O. *J. Nutr.* **96**:375 (1968).

34. Hruza, A. and Fabry, P. *Gerontologia* **1**:279 (1957).

35. Tannenbaum, A. *Cancer Res.* **2**:468 (1942).

36. Silberberg, R. and Silberberg, M. *Can. J. Biochem. Physiol.* **33**:167 (1955).

37. Wynder, E. L. *Cancer Res.* **24**:1235 (1969).

38. Ross, M. H. and Bras, G. *Nature* **250**:263 (1974).

39. Ross, M. H. *Am. J. Clin. Nutr.* **25**:834 (1972).

40. Tannenbaum, A. *Cancer Res.* **4**:673 (1944).

41. King, J. T., Casas, C. B., and Visscher, M. B. *Cancer Res.* **11**:712 (1951).

42. Richter, C. P., Holt, Jr., L. E., and Barelare, Jr., B. *Am. J. Physiol.* **122**:734 (1938).

43. Richter, C. P. and Schmidt, Jr., E. C. H. *Endocrinology* **28**:179 (1941).

44. Mayer, J., Dickie, M. M., Bates, M. W., and Vitale, J. J. *Science* **113**:745 (1951).

45. Donhoffer, S. *Triangle* **4**:233 (1960).

46. Richter, C. P. *Am. J. Physiol.* **115**:155 (1936).

47. Richter, C. P. and Eckert, J. F. *Am. J. Med. Sci.* **198**:9 (1939).

48. Griffiths, Jr., W. *Ann. N.Y. Acad. Sci.* **67**:1 (1956).

49. Richter, C. P. and Barelare, Jr., B. *Endocrinology* **23**:15 (1938).

50. Anliker, J. and Mayer, J. *Am. J. Clin. Nutr.* **5**:148 (1957).

51. Ross, M. H. and Bras, G. *Science,* 1974, in press.

PART 2

Aging in Normal Human Populations

4

Physiologic Changes with Aging

E. J. MASORO

Department of Physiology, The University of Texas Health Science Center at San Antonio, San Antonio, Texas

On the basis of casual observation of old and young people, it would be anticipated that marked physiological changes occur during aging. Surprisingly, therefore, an analysis of the literature on the effects of age on the functioning of the various organ systems leaves this author, at least, with the impression that most physiological activities in normal resting man in the steady state are affected only to a modest extent by aging. In this review of the physiology of organ systems the focus will be on human function, except where definitive data are available only for species other than man. The outstanding fact emerging from this review is the consistent finding of a strikingly more effective response of the young compared to the old to physiologic challenges. Indeed it is such challenges that justify the impression gained from casual observation that marked physiological deterioration occurs with aging. Examples of three such challenges in relation to age will be discussed subsequent to the survey of organ system physiology.

There is much evidence to indicate that a deterioration in function of the cardiovascular system occurs as aging progresses. In Table 1, certain general changes in cardiovascular function with age are presented. The heart rate falls from 25 to 65 years of age. The systolic blood pressure changes little from 25 to 65 years of age, but after the age of 65, systolic blood pressure increases markedly. Diastolic blood pressure significantly increases from 25 to 35 years of age, with little further increase as aging progresses. The resting cardiac output, expressed as the cardiac index, declines at a rate of about 1% per year as the mature adult ages. From these data it is clear that in resting man an increase in total peripheral resistance occurs as aging progresses.

61

Table 1   General Changes in Cardiovascular Function

a. The heart rate of resting man declines from 25
    to 65 years of age (1).
b. Systolic blood pressure of resting man increases
    after 55 years of age (1).
c. Diastolic blood pressure of resting man increases
    from 25 to 35 years of age and changes little thereafter (1).
d. Cardiac index of resting man declines at a rate
    of 1% per year as the mature adult ages (2).
e. Total peripheral resistance of resting man
    increases as aging progresses.

There is a loss of arterial distensibility as man ages (Table 2). This loss in distensibility does not correlate with the extent of atherosclerosis. Indeed, contrary to the marked difference in atherosclerotic severity between Americans and Japanese, loss of aortic distensibility of Americans is not greater than that of the Japanese (4). Therefore, it seems reasonable to conclude that distensibility is an inevitable consequence of aging, whereas atherosclerosis is a disease that tends to occur in the elderly. As a result of this loss of distensibility, the pulse wave velocity increases linearly with age.

Not only does the elastic modulus of the walls of the great arteries increase with age, but these arteries also dilate during aging (Table 2). For the work of the heart to be minimum, it is necessary for the thoracic aorta to present a low impedance to outflow of blood from the heart. An easily distensible tube having a relatively thin wall with a low coefficient of elasticity and hence a low pulse wave velocity will provide this kind of impedance and such is the case with the aorta of young

Table 2   Changes in the Vascular System

a. Arterial distensibility decreases as man ages (3-6).
b. Pulse wave velocity of man increases with age (6).
c. The large arteries of man dilate with age (3).
d. Impedance to left ventricular output of man increases
    after 60 years of age (3).
e. Aortic arch and carotid baroreceptor reflexes of man
    become less sensitive with age (7).

people. However, the aorta of old people is considerably stiffer. In regard to impedance, the stiffness is partly compensated for by the dilatation of the aorta, which causes it to contain a larger volume of blood than the aorta of the young people. Because of this large volume, the heart discharges its stroke volume into the aorta without an excessive rise in pressure and thus a relatively low impedance is maintained. This compensation seems to work fairly well up to 60 years of age, but in people older than 60 the volume increases of aorta no longer compensate for the decreased distensibility. Therefore, in the very old the work of the heart for a given stroke volume is increased.

The baroreceptor reflexes with receptors located in the aortic arch and carotid sinus are important components in the regulation of arterial blood pressure. These reflexes become less sensitive as one ages. This decreased sensitivity is not caused by an altered arterial blood pressure, but seems likely to be due to a reduced sensitivity of the receptors because of a decreased distensibility of the arterial wall in which they are located.

Ideally, three physiologic parameters should be investigated in regard to the effect of age on the functioning of the heart: *(1)* the excitation and conductile properties, *(2)* excitation-contraction coupling, and *(3)* the mechanical response. Electrocardiographic measurements have been the major means of exploring excitation and conduction systems of the human heart. Aging causes marked changes in the electrocardiographic pattern, but the evidence indicates that these changes may be related less to the aging process per se than to the extent of the latent coronary disease (8). Little has been done on the effect of age on the excitation-contraction coupling in cardiac muscle, but some work has been done on the effect of age on the mechanical responses of rat cardiac muscle. It should be noted that the rat cardiac muscle does not show evidence of coronary artery pathology and therefore it is unlikely that the changes described in Table 3 are

Table 3   Cardiac Changes

a.	Duration of contraction, time to peak tension, and relaxation time at maximum tension are prolonged in trabeculae carnae of aged rats (9).
b.	Inotropic responsiveness to catecholamines is decreased in trabeculae carnae of aged rats (10).
c.	Hearts of old rats have a reduced ability to respond to elevated arterial pressure by increasing cardiac work (11).

secondary to coronary heart disease. It has been shown that the duration of contraction, the time to peak tension, and the relaxation time at maximum isometric tension are prolonged in trabeculae carnae obtained from aged rats and that the inotropic responsiveness to catecholamines is decreased in these muscle preparations from aged rats. Moreover, the hearts of old rats have a reduced ability to respond to elevated arterial blood pressure by increasing cardiac work. Although this kind of detailed analysis of the contractile characteristics of cardiac muscle has not been done with human material, there is evidence of a small but significant increase in the left ventricular ejection time as man ages which is independent of changes in heart and blood pressure (12). Moreover, during aging there are cellular changes occurring in cardiac muscle involving neutral fat and lipofuscin deposition (13). It is the lipofuscin deposits that caused the heart of senescence to appear brown in color.

The ventilatory function of the respiratory system also deteriorates with age (Table 4). Maximal breathing capacity is reduced by 40%

Table 4   Respiratory Changes

a.	Maximal breathing capacity and vital capacity of man decline with age (14).
b.	Residual volume and physiological dead space of man increase with age (14, 15).
c.	Elastic recoil of chest-lung system of man decreases with age (16).
d.	Resistance to airflow in the peripheral airways of man increases with age (17).
e.	PO_2 of the arterial blood of man decreases with age (18, 19).

between the ages of 20 and 80 years. Also, there is a diminution in vital capacity and an increase in residual volume with age. The physiological dead space is increased in the elderly, and this increase relates to a change in an alveolar component rather than to an increase in the anatomical dead space.

Many of these changes in pulmonary function are probably attributable to the loss in the elastic recoil that occurs during aging. For example, the increase in the ratio of functional residual capacity to total lung volume observed with aging is most readily explained on this basis. However, in addition to problems secondary to the loss of elastic recoil, there is also an increased resistance to air flow in the peripheral airways of man with increasing age.

The partial pressure of oxygen of arterial blood declines with age. Perhaps the most widely accepted explanation for this decrease in arterial oxygen tension with age is that an alteration occurs in the ventilation/perfusion ratio. However, recent work establishes that no difference can be found in this ratio between young and old subjects (20).

In older subjects, changes of an emphysematous character are often seen even in people who have not been and are not suffering from known clinical respiratory disease (14). Some investigators have applied the name "senile lung" and others "senile emphysema" to these changes. The term "nonobstructive emphysema resulting from age" has also been used. The abundance of abnormal acini encountered in these individuals is quite surprising in view of the absence of respiratory symptoms. Probably the large amount of respiratory reserve normally present affords sufficient protection to prevent overt symptoms. Even though the cysts in this condition are small, they must induce a marked disturbance in the ventilation pattern of the acini, an abnormality that would be further exacerbated by the disruption of capillary circulation. Such changes of course would be consistent with the reduced PO_2 found in the arterial blood of elderly people.

Although under resting steady-state conditions most of the components of the internal environment are maintained at fairly normal levels even at quite advanced ages (21), renal function clearly deteriorates with age (Table 5). The glomerular filtration rate falls as does the renal blood flow. The maximal capacity to secrete PAH (para-aminohippuric acid) and to reabsorb glucose decreases. Most of these functions decrease at the rate of about 0.6% per year in the adult. The ability of man to form either a concentrated or a dilute urine decreases

Table 5   Body Fluid–Renal System

a.	In man the renal blood flow and glomerular filtration rate decline with age (22).
b.	In man, the T_m for glucose and PAH declines with age (22).
c.	In man, the ability to form either a concentrated or dilute urine decreases with age (23).
d.	In rats, there is a decline in number of nephrons with age (22).

Table 6   Gastrointestinal System

---

a.   In man, the ability of parietal cells to secrete HCl
declines with age and in general there is a reduction
in the secretory ability of the digestive glands (21, 24).

b.   In man, xylose absorption is normal until 80 years
of age (26).

c.   In man, calcium absorption decreases with age (27).

---

with age. In the rats there is evidence establishing a loss of nephrons
with age and it is possible that the decreases in renal function in man
are at least in part due to a loss of nephrons.

There is a paucity of physiologic information on the effect of age on
gastrointestinal function (Table 6). However, it has long been known
that the parietal cells of the stomach lose their ability to secrete hydro-
chloric acid as the individual ages. There also appears to be a general
reduction in the secretion of digestive juices in old age. It would seem,
however, that the capacity to digest materials is not markedly reduced
in the aged although there is some evidence from testing with very
large quantities of material that aging causes man to have a relative
insufficiency in his capacity to digest protein (25).

The effect that aging might have on the absorption of foodstuffs has
been tested by using xylose as a marker substance. It is not until man is
over 80 years of age that the intestinal capacity to absorb xylose is
significantly influenced by aging. Calcium absorption, however, does
decrease with age in man.

The motor function of man declines with age (Table 7), the fall in

Table 7   Neuromuscular System

---

a.   In man, motor function declines with age; e.g.,
handgrip strength declines with age (28, 29).

b.   In man, the number of functional motor units
declines with age (30).

c.   In rats, the number of muscle fibers declines with
age (28).

d.   In rats of extreme old age, the speed of contraction
of skeletal muscle decreases as do the myofibrillar and
myosin ATPase activities (31).

e.   In rats, the rate of Ca^{2+} transport by skeletal
muscle sarcoplasmic reticulum increases with age (32).

---

handgrip strength being a case in point. There is, in the case of man at least, a fall in the number of functioning motor units with age. The rat has a decline in number of muscle fibers with age and in extreme old age shows a decrease in speed of contraction and myofibrillar and myosin ATPase activities. The rate of calcium transport by the sarcoplasmic reticulum increases with rat age, which might relate to the muscle dysfunction by making it difficult to obtain sufficient calcium in the myoplasm for the contractile requirements of the actomyosin system.

It is generally believed that with old age there is a decline in the functioning of the central nervous system. However, in many cases, this is due to diseases (e.g., Alzheimer's disease, Parkinson's disease) which are more prevalent in the aged. The question addressed by this review (Table 8) is the extent of deficit in central nervous system function that

Table 8   Nervous System

a.	The slowing in the response to environmental stimuli with age adversely affects human performance (33).
b.	In man and other vertebrates, a loss of neurons with age occurs in some but not in all areas of the CNS (34, 35).
c.	In man, sense organ function is impaired with age, e.g., loss of visual and auditory acuity (36) and loss of olfactory receptors (37).

occurs with aging in the absence of known disease processes. Along this line, it is known that performance in the aged is affected by the slowing of the responses to environmental stimuli. Moreover, in man and in other vertebrates there is a loss of neurons with age in some, but not all, areas of the central nervous system, but it is difficult to know the functional significance of this loss. There is also evidence that the functioning of sense organs is impaired with age. Examples of this are the loss of visual and auditory acuity with age and the morphologic evidence that the number of olfactory receptors markedly declines as man ages.

The idea that aging results from an age-related failure of endocrine glands has been held by many over the years. However, unequivocal experimental data supporting such a thesis have been difficult to come by. In a most recent textbook of endocrinology, Gregerman and Bierman (38) review aging and hormones and summarize the state of the field at this time in a figure reproduced here (Fig. 1). Some specific

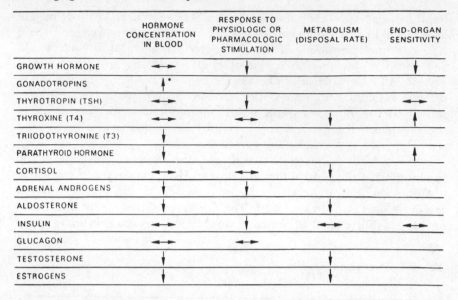

	HORMONE CONCENTRATION IN BLOOD	RESPONSE TO PHYSIOLOGIC OR PHARMACOLOGIC STIMULATION	METABOLISM (DISPOSAL RATE)	END-ORGAN SENSITIVITY
GROWTH HORMONE	←→	↓		↓
GONADOTROPINS	↑ •			
THYROTROPIN (TSH)	←→	↓		←→
THYROXINE (T4)	←→	←→	↑	↑
TRIIODOTHYRONINE (T3)	↓			
PARATHYROID HORMONE	↓			↑
CORTISOL	←→	←→	↓	
ADRENAL ANDROGENS	↓	↓		
ALDOSTERONE	↓		↓	
INSULIN	←→	↓	←→	←→
GLUCAGON	←→	←→		
TESTOSTERONE	↓		↓	
ESTROGENS	↓		↓	

Figure 1.   General summary of endocrine changes with age. From (38).

comments on the information presented in this figure are in order.
When insulin hypoglycemia is used to induce growth hormone secretion, plasma growth hormone levels rise in young and old alike, but the
mean increase in elderly is considerably less than that seen with young
people. Moreover, certain metabolic responses to growth hormone are
blunted in elderly subjects. The ability of the pituitary of elderly subjects to secrete TSH in response to administered thyrotropin-releasing
hormone is decreased in the elderly.

In regard to the thyroid gland, probably the most significant finding
is that blood levels of triiodothyronine (T3) are decreased in elderly
individuals, but the functional significance of this low level of T3 and
relatively normal blood level of thyroxine (T4) remains to be determined. In normal older people there is a small fall in the concentration
of parathyroid hormone in the blood and apparently some heightened
sensitivity in the response of bone to this hormone. It should also be
noted that the blood concentration of testosterone in man and of
estrogens in women decreases with old age.

It has long been known that a decreased glucose tolerance occurs
with age. It does not seem to relate to a decreased sensitivity of the
metabolic system to insulin, but rather to the reduced ability to secrete
insulin in response to challenges. For example, Andres and colleagues
(39) have carried out experiments in nonobese elderly subjects in which

the level of blood sugar used to challenge the organism was controlled at the same level in both young and old. In response to these blood sugar levels, both the early and the late phases of insulin secretion are clearly less in the old subjects compared to the young.

This response of the insulin-secreting system is an example of the general phenomenon of a slowed or lessened ability, or both, to respond to physiologic challenges by the aged. Three such challenges will be briefly discussed: (a) the capacity to carry out vigorous exercise, (b) the response to low environmental PO_2, and (c) the response to a dietary challenge to the acid-base balance.

The maximal oxygen intake ($\dot{V}O_{2max}$) per unit of body weight in response to exercise is a good measure of the capacity to carry out vigorous exercise and is used internationally as a standard of cardio-respiratory fitness. It is equal to the product of the maximum cardiac output and the maximum arteriovenous O_2 difference obtained with highest intensity exercise levels. Cross-sectional data obtained by Dehn and Bruce (40) reveal the average annual decrement in $\dot{V}O_{2\,max}$ with age shown in Fig. 2. Longitudinal data reveal an annual decrement in $\dot{V}O_{2\,max}$ which is significantly greater than that of the cross-sectional studies; moreover there is a stratification according to habitual activity, with the sedentary man experiencing a three times greater decline in

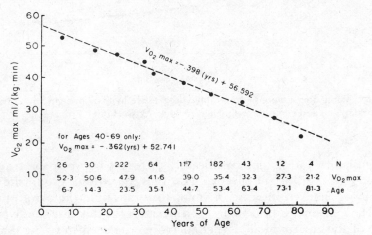

Figure 2. Regression of mean $\dot{V}O_{2max}$ per decade of age for 700 observations in healthy boys and men, recalculated from 17 studies in the literature. Unlike more conventional plots of $\dot{V}O_{2max}$ in liters/min against age, which show an increase with growth and development in childhood and a progressive decline after adolescence, when $\dot{V}O_{2max}$ is corrected for body weight and expressed in ml/(kg·min), there is a fairly uniform decrement throughout life. From (40).

$\dot{V}O_2$ max with age than individuals who habitually participate in weekly running activities. These and similar studies establish the occurrence of a continuous decline in cardiorespiratory function with age. It should be noted that the data described above for individuals in the resting near steady-state conditions did not indicate nearly as great a decline in cardiorespiratory function with age.

Kronenberg and Drage (41) studied the ventilatory response of young (22- to 30-year-old) and old (64- to 73-year-old) men who were free of detectable cardiovascular or pulmonary disease to changing alveolar PO_2 levels (Fig. 3). Clearly, at an alveolar PO_2 of 100 mm Hg

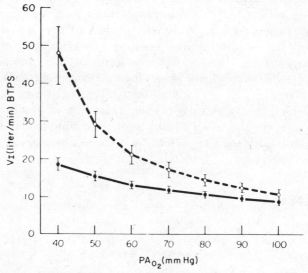

Figure 3. Ventilatory response to isocapnic progressive hypoxia in eight young normal men (broken line) and eight normal men aged 64 to 73 (solid line). From (41).

the ventilatory rate is not significantly different between the two age groups. However, as the alveolar PO_2 falls, the young group shows a much more marked increase in ventilatory rate than the old group of men. Here again we find that a perturbation (in this case the hypoxic nature of the environment) is met far more effectively in young than in old individuals. These data indicate that the older individual is probably more vulnerable both to hypoxic disease states and to high altitudes.

Another example of the relative inability of old people to meet challenges is the differences between young and old in ability to respond to dietary challenges to the acid-base balance. For example, blood pH is not different in young and old people when studied in the resting, steady-state condition. However, Shock (42) reports that the oral administration of 10 grams of ammonium chloride to a young subject will produce a reduction in blood pH of about 0.05 units in 1½ hours with complete recovery by the end of 8 to 10 hours. However, in the 80-year-old this same dose of ammonium chloride will produce a displacement of pH of about 0.15 units and the recovery will require from 24 to 72 hours.

Body composition also changes during aging. Bone loss is a general phenomenon beginning by the fifth decade in both men and women and progressing more than twice as fast in the female than in the male (43). Within broad limits, calcium intake does not relate to this bone loss, since increasing the intake of calcium to above 1.5 grams per day does not seem to be protective in regard to this loss of bone calcium.

It is generally held that there is a loss of lean body mass and increase in the adipose tissue mass with age (44). However, these are complex phenomena and such general statements are not warranted. In this regard, brief mention should be made of two recent research studies in these areas.

First, the work of Lesser and his co-workers (45) on the effects of age on the lean body mass (fatfree mass), which is summarized in Tables 9 and 10, opens to question the concept that the lean body mass declines with age. In their cross-sectional study (Table 9), in agreement with the generally held view, it is evident that the oldest age group of rats did have a somewhat lower lean body mass than the younger rat groups. However in Table 10, in which the data on the longitudinal study of lean body mass with age are presented, no decrease in the lean body mass is found with increasing age of the rats. Further analyses of these

Table 9   Cross-Sectional Study of Rat Age and Lean Body Mass[a]

Age of Rats (days)	Number Studied	Fatfree Mass
345-620	124	558.5 ± 5.0
662-793	67	564.8 ± 8.1
785-918	22	531.1 ± 10.3

[a]From (45).

Table 10   Longitudinal Study of Rat Age and Lean Body Mass of Long-Lived Rats[a]

Age of Rats (days)	Number Studied	Fatfree Mass
345-620	22	516.0 ± 10.4
662-793	22	526.8 ± 9.6
785-918	22	531.1 ± 10.3

[a] From (45).

data led Lesser and his colleagues to conclude that because of selective longevity, animals with lower lean body masses represented the majority of the population in the oldest age group. Thus, the implication drawn from cross-sectional studies that an individual's lean body mass declines with age is not borne out by these rat studies, but rather they indicate that animals with low lean body mass tend to live longer than those who have a large lean body mass. The authors further point out that there is a decline of lean body mass when the animals become diseased, which may account for the intuitive feeling that old people tend to shrink up.

Second, recent work in our laboratory on adipose tissue in relation to age should be mentioned (46). It is generally held that the number of adipose tissue cells (adipocytes) remains constant in the fat depots during the adult life of mammals. It has therefore been concluded that increases in adipose tissue mass that occur during adult life are the result of the increase in the size of the preexisting adipocytes. However, this concept is based primarily on studies of developing rats and young adults. We therefore decided to explore the cellular characteristics of the epididymal fat depot as a function of age through virtually the entire lifespan of males of the inbred Fisher 344 strain of rat.

In Fig. 4, data on the effect of age on the weight of the rat and on the triglyceride content of the epididymal adipose tissue depot are presented. The weight of this population of rats increases until about 52 weeks of age, with a small further increase in the weight occurring during the next 52 weeks of life. The population surviving to 130 weeks of age has a somewhat lower body weight than the population sacrificed at 104 weeks of age. The triglyceride content of the epididymal fat depot, like the body weight, increases markedly with age

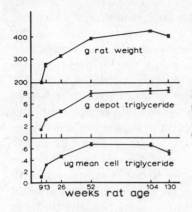

Figure 4. Age, rate weight, epididymal depot triglyceride mass, and fat cell size in male Fisher 344 rats. Plots are mean values ± 1 SEM. From (46).

during the first 52 weeks of life and remains constant for the remainder of the lifespan. The effect of age on the mean size of the adipocyte is also shown in Fig. 4, and the total number of fat cells in the epididymal depot is shown in Fig. 5 along with the mortality characteristics of this strain of rat.

Our results are in agreement with those of others in that from the age of 9 weeks on, increases in the epididymal adipose tissue mass

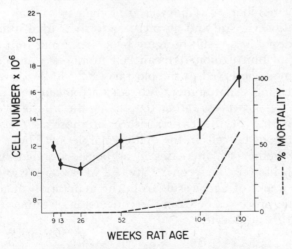

Figure 5. Age and number of fat cells in the epididymal depot. The dotted line represents data from a longevity study on the Fisher 344 strain of rat kept under identical conditions to those used in our work, to be published by C. L. Coleman, A. M. Jonas, H. J. Hoffman, and S. J. Foster, which they have kindly permitted us to use in this graph. The solid line relates to the cell number. Plots are mean values ± 1 SEM. From (46).

primarily result from increases in adipocyte size. However, the chronologic pattern of the changes in size and number of adipocytes in the depot is complex. Between 9 and 13 weeks of life, the number of adipocytes declines significantly while the mean size of these cells increases so markedly that the mass of the epididymal depot increases. From 13 to 26 weeks of age little change occurs in the number of adipocytes in the depot, but the mean size of the adipocytes continues to increase. From 26 to 52 weeks of age both the number of adipocytes in the epididymal depot and their mean size increase. From 52 to 104 weeks of age no change occurs in number of adipocytes or in their size (i.e., during this time period the mass of the depot remains constant). Since the longevity study indicates that about 90% of the rats are still living by 104 weeks of life, it is reasonable to assume that the findings at this point of age are not appreciably influenced by the selective death of rats with unique characteristics in regard to adipose tissue morphology. The population sacrificed at 130 weeks of age has significantly more adipocytes in the epididymal depot, but of a smaller cell size than in the case of the rats of 52 to 104 weeks of age. Since by 130 weeks of age about 40% of the population should have been alive on the basis of the above-cited longevity studies on a comparably maintained population of Fisher 344 strain rats, the following two possibilities exist as reasons for this difference: either 40% of the young rats having a great number of adipocytes are longer lived than others or a decrease in adipocyte size and an increase in their total number takes place in this depot as a result of aging processes. Since only 3% of the aging rat population exhibited mean cell numbers equivalent to the mean cell number observed in the old rats (± 2 SEM), it is most likely that the increasing cell number with very advanced age is a consequence of the aging process rather than being due to the selection of a population because of the earlier death of those animals with the smallest number of fat cells in the epididymal depot. These studies do not indicate whether the increases in adipocyte number during two stages of adult life (i.e., between 26 and 52 weeks of age and between 104 and 130 weeks of age) result from the generation of new adipocytes by mitotic processes or from the conversion of immature preadipocytes to mature adipocytes.

REFERENCES

1.   Shaw, D. J., Rothbaum, D. A., Angell, C. S., and Shock, N. W. *J. Gerontol.* **28:**133 (1973).

2. Guyton, A. C. *Circulatory Physiology: Cardiac Output and Its Regulation.* Saunders, Philadelphia, 1963.

3. Bader, H. *Circ. Res.* **20:**354 (1967).

4. Nakashima, T. and Tanikawa, J. *Angiology* **22:**477 (1971).

5. Mozersky, D. J., Sumner, D. S., Hokanson, D. E., and Strandmess, D. E., Jr. *J. Am. Gerontol. Soc.* **21:**18 (1973).

6. Gozna, E. R., Marble, A. E., Shaw, A., and Holland, J. G. *J. Appl. Physiol.* **36:**407 (1974).

7. Gribbin, B., Pickering, T. G., Sleight, P., and Peto, R. *Circ. Res.* **29:**424 (1971).

8. Simonson, E. *Am. J. Cardiol.* **29:**64 (1972).

9. Weisfeldt, M. L., Loeven, W. A., and Shock, N. W. *Am. J. Physiol.* **220:**1921 (1971).

10. Lakatta, E. G., Gerstenblith, G., Angell, C. S., Shock, N. W., and Weisfeldt, M. L. *Circ. Res.,* in press.

11. Lee, J. C., Karpeles, L. M., and Downing, S. E. *Am. J. Physiol.* **222:**432 (1973).

12. Willems, J. L., Roelandt, J., De Geest, H., Kistloot, H., and Jooseus, J. V. *Circulation* **42:**37 (1970).

13. Burch, G. and Giles, T. *J. Chronic Dis.* **24:** (1971).

14. Pump, K. K. *Chest* **6:**571 (1971).

15. Lifshay, A., Fast, C. W., and Glazier, J. B. *J. Appl. Physiol.* **31:**478 (1971).

16. Turner, J. M., Mead, J., and Wohl, M. *J. Appl. Physiol.* **25:**664 (1968).

17. Niewoehner, D. E. and Kleinerman, J. *J. Appl. Physiol.* **36:**412 (1974).

18. Neufeld, O., Smith, J. R., and Goldman, S. L. *J. Am. Gerontol. Soc.* **21:**4 (1973).

19. Chebotarev, D. F., Korkushko, O. V., and Ivanov, L. A. *J. Gerontol.* **29:**393 (1974).

20. Kronenberg, R. S., Ponto, R. A., and Ebert, R. V. *J. Lab. Clin. Med.* **78:**1008 (1971).

21. Kohn, R. K. *Principles of Mammalian Aging.* Prentice-Hall, Englewood Cliffs, N.J., 1971.

22. Shock, N. W. *Physiologic aspects of aging. J. Am. Diet. Assoc.* **56:**491 (1970).

23. Papper, S. *Geriatrics* **28**(5):83 (1973).

24. Watkin, D. In *Mammalian Protein Metabolism,* Vol. 2 H. N. Munro and J. B. Allison, Eds., Academic, New York, 1964, p. 247.

25. Werner, I. and Hambraeus, L. *Acta Soc. Med. Upsal.* **76:**239 (1970).

26. Guth, P. H. *Am. J. Digest. Dis.* **13:**565 (1968).

27. Bullamore, J. R., Wilkinson, R., Gallagher, J. C., Nordin, B. F. C., and Marshall, P. H. *Lancet* **2:**535 (1970).

28. Gutmann, E. and Hanzlikova, V. *Mech. Age. Dev.* **1:**327 (1973).

29. Clement, F. J. *J. Geront.* **29:**423 (1974).

30. Campbell, M. J., McComas, A. J. and Petito, F. *J. Neurol. Neurosurg. Psychol.* **36:**174 (1973).

31. Syrovy, I. and Gutmann, E. *Exp. Geront.* **5:**31 (1970).

32. Bertrand, H. A., Yu, B. P., and Masoro, E. J. *Mech. Age. Dev.,* in press.

33. Birren, E. J. *The Psychology of Aging.* Prentice-Hall, Englewood Cliffs, N.J., 1964.

34. Brody, H. In *Development and Aging in the Nervous System* M. Rockstein, Ed., Academic, New York, 1973.

35. Wisniewski, H. M. and Terry, R. D. *Prog. Brain Res.* **40:**167 (1974).

36. Webster, I. W. *J. Am. Geriat. Soc.* **22**:13 (1974).

37. Blinkov, S. M. and Glezer, I. I. *The Human Brain in Figures and Tables*. Plenum, New York, 1968.

38. Gregerman, R. I. and Bierman, E. L. In *Textbook of Endrocrinology*. R. H. Williams, Ed. Saunders, Philadelphia, 1974.

39. Andres, R., Pozefsky, T., Swendloff, R. S. and Tobin, J. D. In *Early Diabetes*. R. A. Camerini-Davalos and H. S. Cole, Eds., Academic, New York, 1970, p. 349.

40. Dehn, M. M. and Bruce, R. A. *J. Appl. Physiol.* **33**:805 (1972).

41. Kronenberg, R. S. and Drage, C. W. *J. Clin. Invest.* **52**:1812 (1973).

42. Shock, N. W. In *Papers of Conference in Gerontology*. F. C. Jeffers, Ed., Duke University Council on Gerontology, Durham, N.C., 1962, pp. 123–140.

43. Exton-Smith, A. N. *Am. J. Clin. Nutrition* **25**:853 (1972).

44. Novak, L. P. *J. Geront.* **27**:438 (1972).

45. Lesser, G. T., Deutsch, S., and Markofsky, J. *Am. J. Physiol.* **225**:1472 (1973).

46. Stiles, J. W., Francendese, A. A., and Masoro, E. J. Influence of age on the size and number of fat cells in the epididymal depot, submitted for publication.

5

Protein and Amino Acid Requirements of the Elderly

VERNON R. YOUNG, W. DAVY PERERA, JOERG C. WINTERER, AND NEVIN S. SCRIMSHAW

Department of Nutrition and Food Science and Clinical Research Center, Massachusetts Institute of Technology, Cambridge, Massachusetts

Advances in medical care, coupled with higher living standards, have raised the mean lifespan for populations in the technically developed countries (1). During the past decade or so the number of persons age 65 years or older has continued to increase, both relatively and absolutely, in the United States (2) and Great Britain (3). Hence it may be expected that increased national resources will be devoted to the health and welfare of the aged. If we are to design and implement comprehensive medical care programs for this age group, we must improve our present knowledge of the quantitative aspects of nutrient requirements in the elderly. Unfortunately, nutritional studies in the aged are limited, even though signs of nutritional inadequacy are more common in the elderly than in younger people.

The aging process involves progressive changes in various organs leading to decreased functional ability (4) and the development of disease (5). Together with the physiological and pathological implications of growing old, the health and longevity of elderly people are also influenced by psychologic, economic, sociologic, and physical factors and these, in turn, affect food choices and food habits. All of these

The unpublished studies referred to in this review were supported by National Institute of Health grants AM15892, AM15856, and HD08300. This is publication No. 2538 of the Department of Nutrition and Food Science. The Clinical Research Center is supported through grant No. RR-88 of the General Research Centers Program of the Division of Resources, National Institute of Health.

factors interact in a complex manner that may modify the level of intake of nutrients and the efficiency with which the body utilizes them. It would not be surprising, therefore, to discover that nutrient requirements change with progressive aging in the human subject. However, there is insufficient evidence to evaluate this premise adequately, and neither current United States national (6) nor international (7, 8, 9) dietary allowances have included separate recommendations for the aged. Thus, at present, the planning of nutritionally adequate diets for older people is based largely on the extrapolation of data from studies in healthy young adults.

In this chapter we consider the protein and amino acid needs of elderly subjects by first exploring the possible metabolic basis of these needs, with particular reference to dynamic aspects of whole body protein metabolism during various stages of life. We then examine critically the methods and results of studies concerned with the estimation of essential amino acid and total protein needs. Finally, recommendations are made with respect to dietary protein allowances for the elderly, and critical areas for additional research are considered.

PROTEIN METABOLISM DURING AGING AND ITS RELATION TO PROTEIN NEEDS

The more fundamental aspects of tissue nucleic acid and protein metabolism during aging have been the subject of a number of reviews (1, 10-12) and will not be covered here. However, since the identification and understanding of changes in body and tissue protein metabolism with advancing age should allow a more precise interpretation of data on protein and amino acid requirements and should aid a rational development of nutrient allowances for elderly individuals, some observations on body protein metabolism during aging will be reviewed here.

Body Protein Mass

A major quantitative function of dietary nitrogen and essential amino acids is to furnish substrate required for the maintenance of organ protein synthesis. Therefore, the size and metabolic status of the body protein mass is a factor that will influence the total daily requirement for protein. Adult individuals of differing size but similar age, body composition, sex, and physiological state would be expected to require proportionately differing amounts of protein and essential amino acids

(13). Hence, changes in the distribution and amount of body protein may be considered an initial basis for understanding protein and amino acid needs during the later years of life.

Direct measures of total body protein cannot yet be made with intact subjects although the recently developed procedure of *in vivo* neutron activation analysis (14-16) may provide a reliable, direct estimate of total body nitrogen. However, the use of this procedure is restricted to a few research centers because it requires the use of a cyclotron. To date, there have been no systematic studies of the effects of aging with this method. Therefore, it is necessary to resort to indirect measures, involving densitometric, gasometric, hydrometric, whole body ^{40}K counting, roentgenographic, or anthropometric techniques, to determine the major components of body composition (17-19). Numerous studies have been undertaken to determine body protein in humans and a few of these studies have dealt with the changes in body protein content with advancing years. Cross-sectional as well as longitudinal studies reveal that there is a progressive decline in body potassium (20-22) and a fall in intracellular fluid volume (23, 24) as aging progresses in humans. Because of possible changes in the intracellular concentration of potassium with age, the precise physiological significance of the body potassium loss in the later years is uncertain. Tissues with a high potassium content, such as skeletal muscle, may decrease relative to those with a lower potassium concentration (25, 28), and the relative amount of connective tissue, which contains little potassium (25), may become greater. However, a loss of total body potassium is generally taken to indicate a decrease in total cellular protein mass and this may be due, in large part, to a decrease in skeletal muscle protein mass with age (27-29).

From observations of this kind and other studies of human body composition it is possible to estimate the body N (protein) content at various stages of life. The data, shown in Table 1, indicate that body N increases rapidly from birth during childhood and early maturity, reaching a maximum by about the third decade (22). Thereafter body N decreases more gradually during the later years, with the decline occurring somewhat more rapidly in men than in women (22). These changes have implications for the estimation of dietary protein requirements.

The protein requirement of adults is usually considered to be the dietary intake that is just necessary to achieve a "maintenance" of body nitrogen over relatively short periods. This concept is obviously oversimplified since the chemical composition of the body is in a dynamic state and changes occur in the N content of individual tissues and

Table 1   An Estimate of Changes in Total Body Nitrogen in Man Throughout Life

Age Group	Body Nitrogen	
	g	g/kg body wt
Newborn (full term)[a]	66	19
Child (10 years)[b]	615	19
Adult (25 years)[b]	1320	18
Elderly (65-70 years)[b]	1070	15

[a] Taken from Widdowson and Dickerson (25).
[b] Calculated from the data of Forbes (30) and Forbes and Reina (22), respectively. Estimations made from ^{40}K assuming 68.1 meqK/kg LBM, and from relationships between K, N, and body cell mass (BCM) described by Moore et al. (18).

organs in response to factors such as diet (25), hormonal balance (31), activity patterns (32), and disease (18), in addition to age. However, if this concept is extended to the assessment of protein needs of the elderly, it might be predicted that total protein and possibly individual essential amino acid needs decline with the age-dependent fall in body N mass. A related problem is whether the decline in body N can be modified by diet and whether nutrition may affect the progression of the aging process and result in an increase in mean lifespan. This would be extremely difficult to determine by direct feeding studies in human subjects.

Body and Organ Protein Metabolism

In addition to the total amount of body N, the metabolic status of the individual would be expected to determine the requirements for dietary protein and amino acids. This point is clearly illustrated when the higher protein requirements per unit of body weight for infants and children are compared with those for adults. The difference in protein requirements among these age groups cannot be readily explained by growth rate *per se* or by the daily increment of body N since the latter accounts for only a small percentage of the total body N present at any given time. Therefore, it is worth exploring, at this stage in the discussion, the dynamic aspects of body nitrogen metabolism as a basis for understanding further how old age might influence dietary needs.

Individual Organs

There are currently no published studies of tissue protein synthesis and breakdown in elderly human subjects. However, investigations of plasma albumin degradation rates suggest that they are same in young and old subjects, although the total albumin pool is lower in the elderly (33). The effects of advancing age on protein metabolism in individual organs have been examined in experimental animals. *In vivo* estimates of the rates of disappearance of ^{35}S from proteins of kidney, heart, and skeletal muscle after injection of labeled methionine demonstrated no differences between adult and senescent rats but the rate was higher in the livers of older rats than that obtained in young animals (34). Beauchene and co-workers (35) found an increased incorporation of ^{3}H-isoleucine into liver protein and serum albumin during aging in rats and considered it to be related to the urinary loss of serum proteins that occurs in the aged rat (35-37). Studies on the turnover rates of mitochondrial protein in liver (38, 39) and other tissues (39) have not revealed differences between adult (12 months) and aged (20-24 months) rats, and Chen et al. (40) have concluded that there is no difference in liver total protein synthesis with aging, based on studies with isolated liver microsomes. On the other hand, Hrachovec (41) and Mainwaring (42) observed an age-related decline in protein synthesis by rat and mouse liver microsomes. These diverse findings make it difficult to draw a general picture of the effects of age on the status of liver protein synthesis.

Skeletal muscle mass declines with increasing age and this change is paralleled by a decline in the total RNA concentration in this tissue with aging (43, 44). Additionally, it has been reported that there is a reduction in the protein-synthetic activity of muscle ribosomes *in vitro* with increasing age (45, 46) and a decrease in the proportion of polyribosomes (47). Also, the protein-synthetic capacity of the pH 5 enzyme fraction has been shown to decline in muscle (47), as well as in brain (48), and this may partially account for alterations in tissue protein synthesis with advancing age.

Munro and Gray (49) have concluded from an evaluation of the amount of total RNA in skeletal muscle relative to RNA in the total body that skeletal muscle protein metabolism is proportionately more important in the larger mammalian species than in the smaller species. A similar calculation was made by Young (43) for the rat at different stages of growth. He concluded that the proportion of total body RNA found in the skeletal musculature compared with that in the liver increases throughout the rapid growth phase (Table 2). This finding

Table 2   Total Amounts of RNA in Liver and Skeletal Muscle of the Rat at Different Stages of Growth[a]

Body Weight (g)	Total Organ RNA (mg)		Muscle
	Liver	Muscle	Liver
50	44	27	0.6
100	58	50	0.9
250	104	141	1.4
400	141	127	0.9

[a]Estimates from data of Miller (50) and Young (43).

implies that protein synthesis in muscle represents an increasing proportion of total body protein turnover as growth and development progress. Using this same reasoning, when senescence dominates metabolism and muscle RNA declines, one would predict that muscle protein metabolism would assume a less significant role in total body protein metabolism in the aged organism than in that of young adults.

Plasma Amino Acids

It would be valuable to know the extent to which the decline in muscle mass affects total body amino acid metabolism and dietary requirements for amino acids as aging progresses. For example, depending on the timing of food intake, skeletal muscle exerts a diurnal influence on plasma amino acid levels and may act as a biological reservoir for amino acids consumed in excess of immediate needs (43). Parallel studies in dogs (52) and rats (53) have demonstrated that the liver modifies and regulates the level and pattern of free amino acids in blood plasma during the absorptive phase of the metabolism of protein-containing meals.

Body amino acid metabolism may be explored in man by measuring plasma amino acid levels, and a few investigations have been concerned with these levels in elderly subjects. Wehr and Lewis (54) concluded that 12 of 18 free amino acids measured in plasma samples taken from fasting elderly subjects were elevated, and Armstrong and Stave (55) have reported increased plasma levels of alanine, citrulline, cystine, and tyrosine together with a decrease in serine concentrations as man grows older. However, others have reported reduced levels for most amino acids (56). Thus, the available data do not give rise to a consistent picture. Furthermore, amino acid levels in blood plasma are sensitive to alterations in dietary conditions (57) so that the experimental conditions, including the timing of meals, must be strictly standardized for valid comparisons of plasma amino acid levels among different age groups.

Whole Body N Turnover

Ultimately, studies of protein metabolism at the cellular and organ level should be evaluated in reference to the status of whole body protein metabolism. In this context, Waterlow and Stephen (58) observed that with increased age and body weight, the turnover of body protein decreased in rats (Fig. 1), affecting both liver and muscle (59). Although they did not study rats of advanced age, Yousef and Johnson (60) used ^{75}Se-methionine to study turnover of body protein in rats at 49 days and 600 days. They concluded that there was a marked reduction in total body protein turnover in older rats, but their method is confounded by the effects of amino acid reutilization.

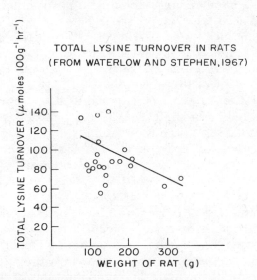

Figure 1. Relationship between total body lysine flux, used as an index of total body protein synthesis, and body weight (age) in rats. Taken from Waterlow and Stephen (58).

As Waterlow (61) points out, it is not sufficiently appreciated that the total body N flux and rates of over-all body protein synthesis and breakdown in human adults are from one to two times greater than the amount of protein normally consumed and three to six times higher than current estimates of the minimum amount of dietary N required to maintain N balance in young adults. This means that there is an extensive reutilization within the body of the amino acids that are released during the course of protein breakdown. If these synthesis and breakdown rates change or the degree of amino acid reutilization is altered as aging progresses, then dietary protein and amino acid requirements can be expected to differ from those determined to be adequate in young adults.

The relatively few available studies of the dynamic and quantitative aspects of body protein metabolism in man provide some insight into changing metabolic needs with increasing age. The evidence suggests that the rate of total body N turnover is twice as high in children, amounting to about 6 g protein/kg body weight/day (62), as in the young adult, whose total body protein synthesis rate approximates 3 g protein/kg/day (63). The relatively high turnover rate in the infant and young child compared with the adult helps to explain a decreased need for protein and essential amino acids as the human passes from infancy to adulthood. Similarly, lower rates of synthesis and breakdown of total body protein in elderly people, if this were determined to be the case, would provide a basis for understanding a possible decline in protein and amino acid needs as aging progresses.

The only published study bearing directly on this aspect of body protein metabolism in man is that of Sharp et al. (64) who studied ^{15}N turnover in four older human subjects with abnormal gastric function. Less ^{15}N was retained after ingestion of ^{15}N-yeast protein by older subjects than by young subjects, and the total body protein synthesis rate was estimated to be equivalent to 0.2 g N/kg/day in the elderly compared with 0.28 g N/kg/day in young subjects (Fig. 2). However, the approach used by Sharp et al. (64) has been criticized on the grounds that the assumptions made in evaluating the ^{15}N data are not valid (63). Furthermore, their method appears to underestimate the actual rate of total body protein synthesis.

Various approaches have been proposed for assessing the quantitative aspects of whole body protein metabolism in human subjects and each approach involves practical and theoretical limitations. Thus, it is not easy to draw an unequivocal conclusion regarding the most suitable model (63) and all of them are oversimplifications of the actual situation in the intact organism. Nevertheless, when the nitrogen turnover

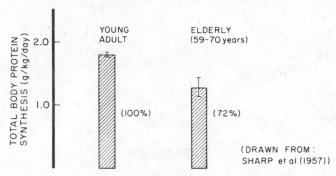

Figure 2.   A comparison of total body protein synthesis rate in young adults and elderly men. Drawn from the data of Sharp et al. (64).

approach to studying whole body protein metabolism is carefully and comparatively applied, it should be possible to obtain useful information about the dynamic aspects of protein metabolism with aging in the human subject.

We have used the Picou and Taylor-Roberts (62) model to study and quantitate whole body N metabolism in the elderly (Fig. 3). The method involves giving a tracer dose of ^{15}N-glycine continuously, or at frequent intervals, during a 30- to 60-hour experimental period. With the administration of the tracer, ^{15}N enrichment of urinary urea increases to achieve a plateau (or quasi-plateau) level. From this level it is possible to estimate the flux (or disposal rate (65)) of N through the metabolic pool and rates of total body protein synthesis and breakdown.

Table 3 compares results that we have obtained using this model in premature infants, young adults, and four elderly women, all studied under comparable experimental conditions. Also included in Table 3 are the data obtained by Picou and Taylor-Roberts (62) in their studies with children 10 to 20 months old who had recovered from protein-energy malnutrition.

During the period of rapid growth and development in children the initially high total body N flux and rate of protein synthesis falls rapidly so that the rates for young adults are approximately one-sixth of those in the newborn. These observations parallel the findings referred to above for rats (58). However, the results summarized in Table 3 also suggest that as the adult years continue the rate of total body

PICOU AND TAYLOR-ROBERTS MODEL*

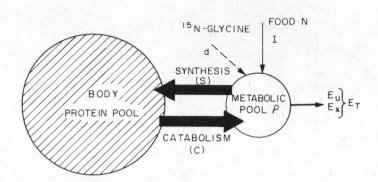

* PICOU AND TAYLOR-ROBERTS (1969) CLIN. SCI. <u>36</u>: 283

d = RATE OF INFUSION OF ^{15}N

e_u = RATE OF EXCRETION OF ^{15}N IN UREA

Q = FLUX OF N THROUGH POOL P

$$F = \frac{e_u}{d} = \frac{E_u}{Q}$$

$$\therefore Q = \frac{E_u}{F} = I + C = S + E_T$$

Figure 3. The constant isotope model of Picou and Taylor-Roberts (62) used for estimating the rate of total body protein synthesis in human subjects. I, C, and S are intake, total body protein breakdown, and synthesis, respectively. E_u, E_x, and E_t are urinary urea, non-urea, and total nitrogen excretions, respectively. Q is the flux (mg N/kg body weight/day) of nitrogen in the metabolic pool, P. F is the fraction of the administered dose (d) of ^{15}N-glycine that is excreted as ^{15}N-urea, or the fraction of total N entering the pool that is excreted as urea N.

protein synthesis, expressed per unit of body weight, gradually falls so that in healthy elderly people it is only 60 to 70% of that observed in young adults.

This fall in the rate of total body protein synthesis with aging parallels the decline, referred to earlier, in total body cell mass. Therefore, additional ways of comparing the rates of total body protein synthesis in young adults and elderly subjects are given in Table 4.

Creatinine excretion has been used as an index of muscle mass (66–68) in children and adults and should have the same meaning in the elderly, even though creatinine clearance is reduced with aging (69). Table 4 shows that total body protein synthesis per gram of

Table 3   Body N Flux and Total Body Protein Synthesis Rate in Humans at Various Ages

Age Group	No. of Studies	N Flux mg N/kg/hr	Total Body Protein Synthesis (g/kg/day)
Newborn (premature)	10	124 ± 46	17.4 ± 9.9
Infant (10-20 months)[a]	4	65 ± 7	6.9 ± 1.1
Young adult	4	26 ± 2	3.0 ± 0.2
Elderly	4	19 ± 2	1.9 ± 0.15

[a] Data for infants taken from Picou and Taylor-Roberts (62). All other values obtained in the authors' laboratories. Mean value ± SD.

Table 4   Total Body Protein Synthesis Rates in Young Adults and Elderly Women

	Young Adult[a] (20–23 years)	Elderly[b] (69-91 years) Actual	Elderly[b] (69-91 years) % of Young Adult
Protein synthesis (per day)			
g/kg body wt	3.0 ± 0.2	1.9 ± 0.2	63
g/kg BCM	6.5 ± 0.7	6.6 ± 1.1	102
g/g creatinine[c]	120 ± 8	168 ± 34	140
g/kcal BMR	0.11 ± 0.01	0.11 ± 0.0	100

[a] Data for three young men and one young woman.
[b] Data for four elderly women.
[c] Per g creatinine excretion per day.
BCM and BMR are body cell mass and basal metabolic rate, respectively.

creatinine excretion is considerably higher in the aged subject than in young adults. Because muscle mass is reduced, the higher turnover per unit of creatinine excretion in the elderly may be interpreted to reflect a greater contribution by the active visceral tissues relative to whole body protein metabolism in the elderly subject.

From these observations it may have been anticipated that total body protein synthesis also would be higher in the elderly when expressed per unit of body cell mass (BCM). However, as shown in Table 4, the rates appear to be similar for the two age groups, and this is also the case when total body protein synthesis rates are related to basal energy expenditure. Therefore, these data suggest that not only is there a probable shift in the distribution of body protein synthesis with advancing age but the rate of muscle protein breakdown and synthesis may decline at the same time. The net result of these concurrent changes is an increase in total body protein synthesis per unit of creatinine with a maintenance of the total body protein synthesis rate when expressed per unit of body cell mass.

This hypothesis of the changes in the quality and quantity of total body protein metabolism can be further supported by comparing urinary N^2-methylhistidine (3-methylhistidine) excretion in young adults and elderly subjects. This unusual amino acid is present in actin of all muscles and in myosin of "white" muscle fibers (70). In rats (71) and man (72, 73) it is quantitatively excreted in the urine and unlike the common amino acids of body proteins it is not reutilized for purposes of protein synthesis (71). Therefore, we have begun to explore the excretion of 3-methylhistidine as a measure of the rate and extent of muscle protein breakdown in human subjects (74).

Preliminary comparative findings on the urinary output of this amino acid in young adults and elderly subjects are given in Table 5. Two conclusions can be drawn from these preliminary data; first, the daily output of 3-methylhistidine is much lower in the elderly than in young adults. This reflects, in part, the lowered muscle mass in elderly subjects. Second, when normalized for differences in creatinine excretion the output of 3-methylhistidine is still quite different between the two age groups. This observation suggests that per unit of muscle mass, the rate of muscle protein breakdown declines appreciably with advanced age.

From these data, one can calculate the total amount of muscle protein breakdown and its contribution to total body protein turnover in young adults and elderly subjects as follows: Asatoor and Armstrong (75) reported a value of about 0.027% for the 3-methylhistidine concentration in mixed proteins of human calf muscle. If this value is

Table 5   Urinary Excretion of 3-Methylhistidine (3 MeH) by Young Men and Elderly Women[a]

Group	Number of Subjects	3-MeH excretion (μmoles)	
		per day	per g creatinine
Young men	2	297,257	137,133
Elderly women	6	79 ± 21	104 ± 15

[a]Unpublished results by L. Haverberg.

representative of the entire skeletal musculature and is applicable to both age groups, then the excretion of 277 μmole of 3-methylhistidine in young adults is roughly equivalent to a daily breakdown of 150 grams of muscle protein. Because the protein synthesis and breakdown rates are essentially equal in adult subjects over short time periods, this breakdown rate is also used as an index of the rate of muscle protein synthesis. By this calculation, therefore, muscle protein accounts for approximately two-thirds of the estimated rate of total body protein synthesis in young men. In contrast, the 3-methylhistidine excretion in the elderly subject is equivalent to about 50 grams of muscle protein breakdown or probably less than 50% of whole body protein breakdown. It must be emphasized that these calculations, based on a few individuals, provide only first approximations of the quantitative nature of the age-dependent redistribution of body protein metabolism with progressive aging in the human subject. However, they support the thesis that muscle protein metabolism accounts for a lower proportion of total body protein turnover in the elderly subject than in younger individuals.

In summary, progressive aging in the human is associated with a decline in the amount of total body protein synthesized daily. This decline is accompanied by a redistribution of protein synthesis within the body so that the visceral tissues make a relatively greater contribution to total body protein synthesis in the elderly than in young adults. From these observations alone, the total protein requirement of the elderly would be predicted to be less per unit of body weight but similar per unit of body cell mass when compared with young adults.

However, it is not yet possible to assess the full nutritional implications of these changes in total body protein metabolism. For instance, the probably greater contribution to total body N metabolism made by liver and other viscera might reduce the need for exogenous amino acids in view of extensive and efficient reutilization of amino acids within the liver cell (76, 77). Furthermore, the decreased need to furnish the peripheral tissues with exogenous amino acids, which must first enter the liver where they may be extensively catabolized, might also serve to reduce the requirement for exogenous sources of nitrogen and essential amino acids. However, these comments are speculative and serve to emphasize the importance of direct metabolic studies to determine the amino acid and protein needs of elderly people.

AMINO ACID REQUIREMENTS

Adequate protein nutrition depends on an exogenous supply of both essential amino acids and nonspecific nitrogen. A number of published reviews (78-80) have also dealt with this topic, and Irwin and Hegsted (81) have recently summarized most of the published studies on the essential amino acid needs in human subjects of all ages.

Nitrogen Balance Studies

Nitrogen balance has been the major criterion used to assess the minimal requirements for the essential amino acid needs in older children (82) and adult men and women (83). In the case of infants body weight gain has also been used (84). These studies reveal a wide variation in the needs for individual essential amino acids among subjects of similar age and body weight. The variation encountered is presumably due both to biological variation among individuals and to experimental and analytical error. It is also worth noting that the nitrogen balance data have been interpreted in different ways for purposes of assessing the minimal needs for the individual essential amino acids. Rose (83) considered that the minimum requirement was met by the lowest level of intake of the amino acid that would maintain a "distinctly positive" N balance. On the other hand, Leverton and co-workers (85) chose the "equilibrium zone," defined as being within 5% of N equilibrium, as the end point in their assessment of the minimum essential amino acid needs in adult women. Differences such as these in the interpretation of N balance data undoubtedly account for some of the variation between laboratories in the reported minimum requirements for the specific essential amino acids.

Compared with studies on the amino acid requirements of young adults there have been few definitive studies of the essential amino acid requirements in the elderly (Table 6). Tuttle, Swendseid and colleagues conducted a series of studies of the essential amino acid requirements of elderly men. In their first study, with five men aged 52 to 68 years, Tuttle et al. (86) concluded that elderly subjects may have a higher requirement for one or more of the essential amino acids than younger persons. A second study by these investigators (87) in subjects over 50 years of age suggested that the requirements of one or more essential amino acids may also increase as the total dietary nitrogen intake rises. Seven subjects maintained nitrogen equilibrium on a diet providing 7 g total nitrogen and an intake of essential amino acids equivalent to 39 g egg protein. Increasing the total nitrogen intake to 15 g/day by addition of glycine and diammonium citrate to the diet caused seven of eight subjects to go into negative nitrogen balance. In further studies (88) the source of the dietary "nonspecific nitrogen" was found to be important in maintaining adequate protein nutrition in elderly subjects since nitrogen retention was higher when a mixture of nonessential amino acids was used in place of glycine as the source of supplemental nitrogen.

Two differing conclusions have been drawn for the minimal methio-

Table 6   Some Mean Estimates of Requirements for Essential Amino Acids in the Elderly Compared with Values for Young Adults

Amino Acid	Number of Subjects	Age (Years)	Mean Requirement (mg/kg/day)	Reference
Elderly				
Methionine	4	64 ± 6	46	(89)
Lysine	4	59 ± 5	30	(89)
Tryptophan	14	73 ± 5	2	(118)
Threonine	11	72 ± 5	8	(116)
Young adult				
S-Amino acid			13	(80)
Lysine			10	(80)
Tryptophan			3	(114)
Threonine			7	(116)

nine requirements of the elderly. Tuttle et al. (89) gave a synthetic L-amino acid mixture, patterned as in egg protein, to six males, 58 to 73 years of age. Total nitrogen intake was 7 g/day. Four subjects receiving no cystine required 2.4, 2.7, 3.0, and 3.0 g, respectively, to achieve nitrogen equilibrium. Two other subjects receiving only small amounts of cystine (less than 50 mg) required greater than 2.1 g daily. These values for the S-amino acid needs of the elderly are considerably *higher* than for the young adult (Table 6). Tuttle et al. (89) also further suggest that the requirement for lysine is higher for the elderly. In contrast with these findings, six black men, 65 to 84 years, studied by Watts and co-workers (90) required *lower* intakes of the sulfur-containing amino acids to achieve N balance. In the Watts study, the dietary essential amino acids simulated the 1965 FAO study (91), and milk patterns were provided as a synthetic mixture, with a total N intake of 10 g/day. With the milk pattern, body N equilibrium was achieved with an intake of 600 mg sulfur-containing amino acids for one subject, 580 mg for two subjects, 450 mg for two subjects, and 287 mg for the remaining subject. These values are similar to those determined for young adults (83).

The apparently contradictory conclusions arising from the studies by Tuttle et al. and Watts et al. may be due simply to wide individual variation and experimental errors in the use of the nitrogen balance technique, or differences in composition of the basal diet and amino acid mixtures used may also be factors. It is also uncertain whether a higher requirement for methionine in elderly men, as reported by Tuttle et al. (89), is due to an increased need for this amino acid or whether, if true, it is due to a reduced efficiency of conversion of methionine to cystine in older individuals. The experimental diet used by Tuttle et al. (89) did not contain significant amounts of cystine and a report by Gaull et al. (92) suggests that the newborn infant has a lower capacity to convert methionine to cystine than the young adult. Whether aging influences the efficiency of conversion of methionine to cystine remains to be established.

The Plasma Amino Acid Approach for Quantitating Essential Amino Acid Requirements in Elderly Subjects

As an alternative to the N balance technique for estimating amino acid requirements, we have explored a new approach that is based on measurement of the concentration of free amino acids in blood plasma. The relationships between the concentration of free amino acids in blood plasma and dietary amino acid intake have been the subject of reviews (57, 93, 94), and studies in the chick (95, 96), rat (97, 98), pig (99), and in man (100-102) have established that a reduced concentration of an essential amino acid in plasma reflects a deficient level of that amino acid in the diet. Therefore, measurements of plasma amino acid concentrations have been proposed for the purpose of evaluating the quality of the dietary protein (100, 103-105). The pattern of amino acids in plasma, as well as the level of a specific essential amino acid in plasma, correlate with the ability of the dietary protein to support growth in experimental animals (57, 93). In this case determination of plasma amino acid levels should allow a prediction of dietary amino acid needs in man at various ages.

Studies in the chick (106), rat (107-110), pig (111, 112), and sheep (113) have demonstrated that, under well-defined conditions, a predictable relationship exists between the plasma concentration of the test amino acid and the intake of the amino acid in relation to the minimum requirement. This relationship is schematically depicted in Fig. 4 and we have explored this approach for assessing the minimum requirements for tryptophan (114), valine (115), and threonine (116) in young adults.

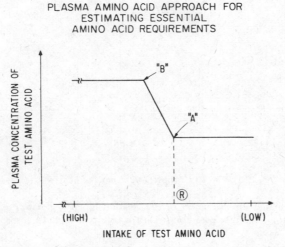

PLASMA AMINO ACID APPROACH FOR
ESTIMATING ESSENTIAL
AMINO ACID REQUIREMENTS

Figure 4. Schematic relationship between the plasma concentration of an essential amino acid, the intake of the amino acid, and the minimum physiological requirement for that amino acid. This figure is based on an interpretation of studies of the plasma amino acid responses in young men (114–118). The "high" level of intake approximates the level of amino acid that is usually consumed. Point A represents the lower breakpoint and point B corresponds to the upper breakpoint.

As shown in Fig. 5, plasma total tryptophan concentration in young men remains at a low and constant level until the minimum requirement level (as judged from N balance data) is exceeded. Beyond this level of intake the concentration of plasma tryptophan increases linearly with increments in dietary tryptophan until a second plateau is reached. This latter intake level is about 2 to 3 times the minimum requirement level. From these results it is suggested that the tryptophan requirement of young adult men is close to 3 mg/kg/day. In a similar study (117) with five mentally retarded children age 6 to 12 years, the shape of the plasma tryptophan response curve was essentially the same as that for young adults, but the lower breakpoint occurred at a tryptophan intake of 4 mg/kg/day for this younger age group.

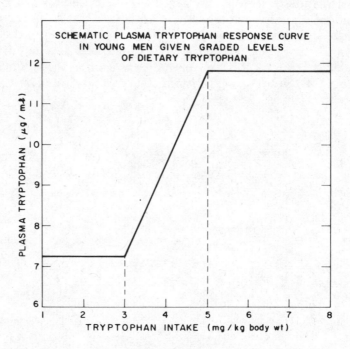

Figure 5. Schematic representation of the relationship between tryptophan in blood plasma and tryptophan intake based on studies in young men (114).

To explore further the nature and significance of the plasma amino acid response curve for estimating human amino acid needs we have extended our studies to older subjects (116, 118) (a) to determine whether the shape of the response curve was affected by increasing age and (b) to estimate the essential amino acid needs in elderly people by the identical method applied in young adult subjects. In the first of the studies (118) with 14 elderly subjects, 73 ± 5 years old, the relationships between plasma tryptophan concentration, tryptophan intake, and tryptophan requirement were examined. The experimental diet was based on an L-amino acid mixture, patterned as in egg protein, and provided N equivalent to approximately 0.5 g protein/kg body weight/day. Plasma tryptophan concentration decreased as tryptophan intake was reduced to the 2 mg/kg/day level (Fig. 6). Thereafter, it remained relatively constant as the intake level was reduced further, indicating a tryptophan requirement in healthy, elderly subjects of approximately 2 mg/kg body weight/day. This is lower than the value of 3 mg/kg determined in young men (114) by the same procedure (Table 6).

The same approach has been used to determine the threonine requirement in elderly subjects (116). Plasma threonine levels decreased with graded reductions in threonine intake until the intake reached a

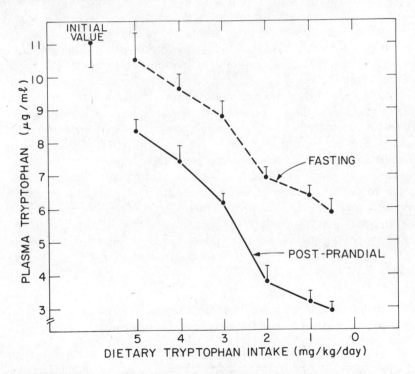

Figure 6. Plasma tryptophan response curve in elderly people consuming graded intakes of dietary tryptophan (116).

level of close to 6 mg/kg/day. A statistical evaluation of the plasma data for each individual subject provided the estimate of threonine requirements which may be compared with values for young adults and elderly, as summarized in Table 6. These results, based on plasma amino acid levels rather than data derived from short-term N balances which are more prone to significant errors, show that the daily threonine requirement of elderly women, expressed per unit of body weight, is the same as for young men. However, this means that the threonine requirement per unit of total body protein increases with age because lean body mass is reduced and the proportion of body fat increased in the older subject, as discussed above. Preliminary data obtained so far with the plasma valine response curve in elderly people suggest that the valine requirement also may be higher per unit of cell mass in the elderly than in young adults.

The studies we have carried out to date have involved mainly females and are still limited in number, so that firm conclusions regarding the comparative essential amino acid needs of healthy elderly individuals cannot be made. However, our findings to date suggest that the requirements for essential amino acids *per unit of body cell mass* may be higher than they are for young adults. This conclusion assumes that the young adult and the elderly subject respond with a similar quantitative and time-dependent response to inadequate intakes of a specific essential amino acid. However, this may not be true in view of the observations by Adelman and co-workers (12) showing that in older animals the metabolic response to hormonal treatment, as measured by changes in liver enzyme activity, is delayed in the aged organism. Their findings not only emphasize the need for fundamental studies of the aging process but also point to the potential value of such studies in developing a more rational and precise comparative nutritional approach to the evaluation of essential amino acid needs, as well as the need for total dietary protein. Thus, the metabolic equivalence of experimental dietary periods of a given duration in young and older people receiving apparently inadequate intakes of essential amino acids may be identified more precisely through studies of the kind carried out by Adelman et al. (12).

The Nutritional Significance of the Plasma Amino Acid Response Curve in Estimating Needs for Essential Amino Acids

Studies in growing experimental animals (106, 108) have shown that the concentration of a specific essential amino acid in plasma remains low and constant until the requirement for that amino acid is met. At about this level of intake the plasma concentration begins to rise in response to further increases in the intake of the amino acid. Hence, in our studies on the plasma amino acid approach for assessing human requirements we have interpreted the lower "breakpoint" on the response curve with human subjects to occur at that intake of the amino acid which just meets the minimum physiological requirement (see Fig. 6). Thus, our definition is operational and the significance of the lower breakpoint is based on a broad extrapolation of observations from experimental animal studies. The additional support for this choice is that the breakpoints in the plasma tryptophan, valine, and threonine response curves in young adults occur at intakes of the amino acids that correspond with the minimum levels, reported earlier by Rose (83), found to be sufficient to maintain N balance in this age group.

However, it could also be argued that the minimum physiological requirement for the amino acid is actually higher than that estimated from the lower breakpoint values on the plasma amino acid response curve. In fact, in consideration of the "idealized" plasma amino acid response curve, shown in Fig. 6, the requirement may be met at an intake that corresponds to the upper breakpoint on the response curve or at an intake that is intermediate between those bounded by the lower and upper breakpoints. Although we have not explored in any detail the plasma amino acid response curve in the region of the upper breakpoint, the summary given in Table 7 is an attempt to define the

Table 7   Estimated Mean Intakes of Essential Amino Acids Required to Maintain Plasma Levels at the Lower and Upper Breakpoints in Young Men[a]

	Intake (mg/kg/day)		Intake from
Amino Acid	lower breakpoint	upper breakpoint	94 mg N/kg/day of egg protein
Tryptophan	3	5-6	10
Threonine	7	> 18 < 30	30
Leucine	22	< 40	50
Valine	16	> 18 < 42	42

[a]Based on data in (114), (115), (116), (118), and unpublished results for leucine.

minimum levels of intake of the amino acids that would be required to support a plasma concentration at the upper plateau value. These levels are compared with the intakes of amino acids provided by egg protein at a level that is very close to the minimum physiological requirement for good quality protein in young men. It may be significant that for tryptophan, threonine, and leucine the upper breakpoint occurred at approximately twice the level of intake that corresponded to the lower breakpoint. Although the nutritional and health significance of this observation is not clear, it may mean that the essential amino acid requirements of adult individuals are considerably higher than the current estimates suggest as being sufficient to maintain adequate protein nutritional status. Also Weller and co-workers (119) have concluded that the requirement for one or more of the essential amino acids in young men, is more than one-third below the needs established by Rose. Additional research is clearly needed to explore this area, particularly since the long-term health significance of estimated amino acid requirements remains to be established.

A further point arising from our comparative studies in young adults and elderly people is that the optimal pattern of essential amino acid requirements may change during old age. It has been assumed that dietary protein quality is the same for young adults and elderly subjects but there are no satisfactory data to support or reject this assumption.

Studies of N utilization using various proportionality patterns of amino acids have been conducted in adult man with a view to determining the importance of dietary amino acid balance in human protein nutrition (120). Swendseid et al. (121, 122) found that N utilization was similar when amino acids were given at isonitrogenous levels from egg or from the 1957 FAO reference patterns. The latter pattern was developed according to the reported requirements for amino acids in man. The studies of Leverton and Steel (123) and of Watts et al. (124) are in general agreement with those of Swendseid and co-workers, but others (125) observed that the 1957 FAO pattern was inferior to various food protein patterns. Recently, Weller et al. (119) reported that the egg pattern, with tryptophan intake set at 330 mg/day and a total N intake of 7 g daily in adult men, was superior to that of the Rose pattern (83), from which the 1957 FAO reference pattern was largely derived.

The effects of excess intakes of the individual essential amino acids have been studied by Clark and co-workers (126), who evaluated the effects of relatively high intakes of methionine, leucine, and valine. They found that dietary N utilization was not significantly depressed by high intakes of each of these amino acids when the intakes of the other essential amino acids and of total dietary N were adequate. However, when the intake of one or more of the essential amino acids was marginal, relatively small changes in the proportion and level of intake of an amino acid resulted in either distinctly beneficial or detrimental effects of N balance (127).

Additional examples of the adverse effects of amino acid disproportions have been reported for man (128, 129). Furthermore, the effects may vary with the particular essential amino acid as demonstrated by Sugahara et al. (130) in their studies with young chicks. Finally, some investigators have claimed that the source and level of nonspecific nitrogen intake affects the over-all utilization of dietary N (131) and influences the requirement for essential amino acids (132, 133).

Although the foregoing supports the view that an intricate balance exists among the essential amino acids, the available data are largely of qualitative significance; the quantitative extent to which the utilization of the individual amino acids is affected by changes in the pattern and level of amino acid intake cannot yet be stated except in a few cases (128). It is not known whether elderly subjects are more or less sensitive to these changes than young adults.

These considerations indicate that the balance and absolute intake of the essential amino acids provided by the experimental diets probably affect the minimum amount of the test amino acid that is found to be required for maintenance of N equilibrium.

PROTEIN REQUIREMENTS

Much of the published data in this area have been compiled in a recent monograph by Irwin and Hegsted (134), which supplements a number of detailed reviews on protein requirements in the elderly (78-80).

Approaches and Methods

As discussed above, the maintenance of body cell mass (BCM) over short periods in young adults and elderly subjects or the achievement of a given rate of BCM gain in the growing child is usually assumed to indicate an adequate protein nutritional status. Thus, the more extensive data on the protein needs of the elderly have been derived from metabolic N balance studies. Additionally, surveys of dietary protein intake have been used to supplement information on protein requirements of various age groups, including the elderly.

The two major N balance approaches have been followed for estimating the minimum physiological needs for total protein. They are (a) the factorial approach, and (b) a measure of N intake required to just maintain body N balance. In young infants, growth rate has been used for determining the minimum physiological requirement.

Factorial Method

In this approach the losses of "obligatory" N via urine and feces are measured and summated with additional corrections for N losses through the integument and other minor routes. In the case of the growing child a further allowance is made for the increment in total body N.

The aim of the method is to determine the total nitrogen loss occurring from the body when the subject receives a protein-free but otherwise adequate diet. The loss is measured after a period of stabilization, and is taken to represent an obligatory loss which is, therefore, the minimum nitrogen output consistent with a normal healthy state. The minimum dietary protein requirement is then computed to be that amount of good quality protein necessary to balance this endogenous loss. The obligatory nitrogen losses occur through three principal routes, urine, feces, and skin, as well as through such minor routes as menstruation and seminal ejaculation, and still lesser losses occur through saliva, expectorated sputum, nasal secretions, and blood losses from trivial wounds. Nitrogen losses occurring from the skin in the form of desquamated cells, hair, and nails, and via sweat constitute the integumental fraction.

Obligatory urine and fecal N losses in adults are measured after a suitable period of stabilization on a protein-free diet (Fig. 7). Nitrogen losses through the integument are far more difficult to measure. Nevertheless, careful studies have quantitated integumental N losses under conditions of a protein-free diet (135, 136). With a usual dietary protein intake the cutaneous and other minor N losses are estimated to average about 5 mg N/kg body weight in adult men (9). Kraut and Müller-Wecker (137) have estimated the integumental losses of N in a few women to be about 3.6 mg N/kg body weight under normal dietary conditions. Conditions which lead to profuse sweating may result in higher N losses through sweat especially in subjects unaccustomed to living and working in hot climates (134).

The major assumption made in applying the factorial approach is that losses of N measured with a protein-free intake can be used to predict the N losses occurring when diet N intake just meets the needs for high quality protein to maintain body N content. Previously it was also assumed that both essential amino acids and total N of hen's egg protein and lactalbumin are completely utilized for purposes of protein

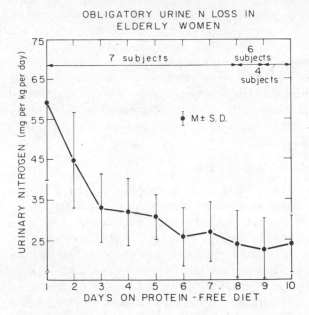

Figure 7. Change in urinary nitrogen excretion during a 10-day period of a protein-free diet in elderly women.

synthesis and other functionally important N-containing compounds. However, recent reports (138-141) have shown for both growing children and adults that this assumption is no longer valid. In fact, more high quality protein is required to achieve N equilibrium than predicted by the summated obligatory losses alone. How much more protein is needed is still uncertain. In the case of adults, two recent studies with American males (138, 139) suggest about 30% more, and the studies of Inoue et al. (140) in young Japanese male subjects indicate as much as a 100% increase above that predicted from the summated losses of obligatory N. For children, the data are also limited but suggest approximately a 30% difference between the factorially derived figure and the amount of high quality dietary protein N actually required for meeting the needs for maximum N retention (141).

With these findings on the relationships between the minimum N intake required to achieve balance and the known magnitude of the total obligatory N losses, the factorial method offers a means of estimating minimum protein needs of various weight and age groups. This approach was adopted by the United States Food and Nutrition Board (6) and FAO/WHO (9) in arriving at recent recommendations for dietary protein. Direct estimates of the obligatory N losses in elderly subjects are discussed below but it should be pointed out here that there are no statistically reliable data that provide sufficient knowledge of the covariance between obligatory N losses and the minimum protein needs of healthy subjects. Hence, further work is needed to establish the relationships between obligatory N losses and the protein needs of individual subjects if the factorial method is to be used reliably for predicting protein needs for various age and weight groups and physiological states.

The N Balance Response Method

In this approach the N balance response to graded intakes of protein within the region of maintenance N intake is determined. In theory, this method is a more direct way of estimating protein needs, but it suffers from the following limitations of the N balance technique. (1) Maintenance N balance does not necessarily reflect maintenance of a steady-state level of protein nutritional status because it does not reveal alterations in the internal distribution of tissue protein metabolism and changes in cell function. (2) Body N balance can be achieved over a wide range of protein intake during short-term periods and, thus, the criterion of N equilibrium as a measure of adequacy may be insufficient, when considered alone, to arrive at a reliable estimate of the minimum protein need. (3) It is difficult to quantitate all of the routes of N loss but they all are important for purposes of estimating N equilibrium or positive balance. Furthermore, if the rate of N loss through one route changes, adjustments may be needed in the losses of N through another. Thus, unless all routes of N loss are measured, erroneous conclusions may be drawn from apparent N balance values. (4) Errors in the technique are larger when the diet is higher in N, and tend to be cumulative and so frequently overestimate true N balance. (5) Various factors other than the protein intake of the diet affect the sensitivity and absolute value of the N balances. These must be considered in evaluating conclusions drawn from N balance results. Such factors as level of energy intake and prior nutritional state of the subject as well as the length of the dietary period affect the results.

In spite of these limitations, N balance measures can provide useful information on the comparative protein needs of elderly human subjects if suitable experimental conditions are chosen and applied in the same way in parallel studies with young adults.

Dietary Surveys

An evaluation of food consumption data of healthy populations formed the basis of some of the earliest assessments of human protein requirements. The invasion of the privacy of a household and barriers imposed by prestige values attached to amounts and types of foods consumed by people, among other factors, make the collection of accurate and reliable estimates of the usual level of food consumption by individuals a difficult task. The actual weighing of foodstuffs prepared for cooking, coupled with a verification of consumption, is the more precise of the approaches, and this can provide useful information about the general level of protein intake for a population group. This approach has been applied to obtain estimates of the levels of protein consumption that are consistent with the absence of biochemical or clinical nutritional disease. However, such estimates do not provide an index of the minimum amount required for maintenance of adequate protein nutritional status. The use of the dietary survey approach will not be discussed further.

Obligatory N Losses and the Factorial Estimation of Protein Needs in the Elderly

The major route of obligatory N loss in adult man is through the urine. For comparative purposes Table 8 summarizes our results obtained previously in young adult men (13) together with those for seven elderly women studied recently at the Massachusetts Institute of Technology Clinical Research Center. Although comparative studies of endogenous nitrogen metabolism in young adults and in elderly subjects who have been studied under essentially identical experimental conditions are confined to our own studies, for purposes of further evaluation we have included in Table 8 the data of Smith and Bricker (142) based on studies with 25 college women.

Obligatory urinary N excretion in healthy elderly women is markedly lower than that found for young men (13, 138, 144) but is comparable to the values of Bricker and Smith (142) and Hawley et al. (145) obtained for young women. Hence, for the same body weight, the total daily obligatory urinary N loss appears to be similar in young and old women. However, it should be mentioned that Murlin et al. (146) found only a trivial difference between urinary N excretion in 28 men and 7 women but their results may be partly confounded by the relatively short experimental diet periods they employed.

Because body composition changes with advancing age it is worthwhile to consider the metabolic implications of the apparently similar values for obligatory urine N losses with advancing age in women, as suggested from the comparisons given in Table 8. For this reason N loss has also been expressed in relation to body cell mass, basal energy expenditure, and creatinine excretion.

Table 8   Obligatory Urinary Nitrogen Losses in Young Adults and Elderly Women

	Young Adults		Elderly Women
	Men[a]	Women[b]	
Urine nitrogen			
mg/kg/day	37.2 ± 5.5	25.2 ± 3.3	24.8 ± 6.5
mg/kg BCM/day[c]	76.8 ± 12.5	62 ± 10	89.0 ± 20.1
mg/basal kcal	1.77 ± 0.30	1.14 ± 0.11	1.44 ± 0.14
g/g creatinine	1.58 ± 0.22	1.29 ± 0.11	2.14 ± 0.32
g/day	2.69 ± 0.48	1.45 ± 0.15	1.44 ± 0.23
Creatinine (g/day)	1.72 ± 0.24	1.13 ± 0.13	0.68 ± 0.09

[a] Data from Scrimshaw et al. (13).
[b] Taken and calculated from Bricker and Smith (142).
[c] BCM measured by whole body ^{40}K in men and elderly women. For young women BCM estimated, using body height, from prediction equations derived by Forbes (143).

Mean obligatory urinary N output per unit of body cell mass is higher in elderly women than in younger men and women. This difference may reflect the redistribution of total body protein synthesis with age, as discussed earlier, or it may mean that elderly subjects adapt less efficiently to a protein-free diet than younger subjects. Furthermore, endogenous N output per unit of creatinine would be expected to be higher in elderly subjects, and this is supported by the comparative data shown in Table 9. Whether there is a real change in the obligatory N loss per unit of basal energy expenditure with increased age is less certain. Our findings with young men suggest a higher rate of N excretion per basal kcal than for elderly women. However, from other studies with young men (138) there is no clear indication that the obligatory urine N loss, when expressed in relation to basal metabolism, changes substantially with increasing age in the adult human subject.

Similar comparisons may also be made for obligatory fecal N output, and these estimates are given in Table 9. The reported values for adult males range from 9 to 23 mg N/kg body weight, and the 1973 FAO/WHO Expert Group on Protein and Energy Requirements (9) chose a value of 12 mg N/kg as being a weighted mean for young men. The value of 8.7 mg N/kg for obligatory fecal N loss in young women reported by Bricker and Smith (142) closely compares with a mean value of 9.8 mg N/kg/day for the elderly women. Thus, on the basis of these limited data for healthy elderly subjects the obligatory fecal N loss is concluded to be similar to that for young adults.

Total obligatory N losses for adult men have also been computed, as shown in Table 9, and compared with the values obtained with elderly women. From this comparison the total obligatory nitrogen loss in elderly women is similar to that for younger women and lower than the values generally obtained with young men (13, 138, 146). However, our estimate for elderly women is somewhat lower than the mean value of 49 mg N/kg for total obligatory N loss assumed for young women by the 1973 FAO/WHO Expert Group (9). This difference is largely because the Group applied the same value to adults of both sexes for

Table 9   Total Obligatory N Losses[a] and Calculated Safe Practical Allowance for Protein in Young Adults and Elderly Women

	Young Women			Elderly Women
	Men	Women	1973 FAO/WHO (Female)	
Obligatory fecal N (mg/kg/day)	8.8 ± 2.1	8.7 ± 1.6		9.8 ± 3.1
Total obligatory N[b] (mg/kg/day)	51	38	49	40
Estimated requirement (mg/kg/day) +30% for individual variability	66	51	64	52
+30% for efficiency of N utilization	86	66	83	67
Safe practical allowance g protein/kg/day	0.54	0.41	0.52	0.42

[a] Data for elderly women and young adults based on (13) and (142).
[b] Includes 5 mg N/kg/day for integumental and other minor losses (9).

obligatory urinary N losses. From these values a prediction can now be made of the minimum protein needs of adult subjects.

First, in order to cover the total nitrogen (protein) needs for nearly all members of a population group it is necessary to account for variability in N losses among individuals. Based on studies in a large number of adult men a value of 15% has been taken as an estimate of the coefficient of variation in the adult population (9). Thus, a value of 30% above average total obligatory N losses should cover the total N losses for the majority of individuals. Our results with a limited number of healthy elderly women indicate a coefficient of variation of approximately 20%, or a variance similar to that for young adults.

Second, as discussed earlier, it is now known that the factorial summation of obligatory N losses underestimates actual nitrogen needs from whole-egg protein for maintenance. Therefore, the total obligatory nitrogen losses must be increased by a further 30% to obtain the final estimation of the minimum physiological N requirement. These two adjustments, one for individual variation and the other taking into account the inefficiency of dietary N utilization at requirement levels of N intake, have been used to compute the minimum physiological requirement for good quality protein in young adults and elderly women. The estimations are also given in Table 9.

If we use the factorial approach our new data on endogenous N metabolism in elderly people suggest that 0.42 g protein (N × 6.25)/kg/day would be a safe practical allowance for healthy elderly women. This compares with the 1973 FAO/WHO (9) values of 0.57 g and 0.52 g protein/kg/day for healthy young men and women, respectively. There are no comparable data yet available to provide a similar practical allowance for healthy elderly men.

Nitrogen Balance Response and Minimum Protein Needs in the Elderly

In addition to the factorial approach discussed in the preceding section, the minimum physiological needs for dietary protein may be directly determined from the N balance response to graded protein intakes. Watkin (147) has carefully reviewed this topic and has discussed the factors that may account for the lack of agreement among the various studies, of which there are many. Few studies, however, allow definitive conclusions to be drawn concerning the minimum protein needs of older people. Table 10 summarizes some of the N balance studies and conclusions drawn from them. Some investigators (151) concluded that the needs for protein were higher in the elderly

Table 10   Some Studies on N Balance and Protein Needs in the Elderly

Estimate and Conclusion	Remarks	Reference
N equilibrium in 7 of 8 women at 0.7 and 1.0 g protein/kg Dietary standards adequate	Healthy women, 52-74 years	(148)
Good nutritional state maintained at 54 ± 5 g protein	N balance assessed from diet records 20 women, 68-88 years	(149)
Protein needs not different from younger adults	Review of studies with older men and women in a mental hospital	(150)
No evidence of qualitative or quantitative changes with age	Balance studies in healthy old men	(147)
Elderly require 0.7 g protein/kg/day	4 men, 69–76 years, poorly nourished subjects	(151)
Protein requirement for elderly women may be 20–30% less than for young women	9 women, 66–94 years old. Maintained health at self chosen intakes	(152)

than in young adults, whereas others (147, 149, 150) considered that there were no substantial differences between the requirements for protein in young and old adults. On the other hand, Albanese et al. (152) suggested from their earlier studies that the protein requirement may be lower for elderly women than intakes recommended for young sedentary women.

A number of the studies referred to in Table 10, as well as others reviewed by Watkin (147) and Irwin and Hegsted (134), were not based on precise N balance determinations, and, furthermore, conclusions were made in conjunction with the views on the estimated protein needs of younger adults when these earlier studies were carried out. Also, the levels of protein intake tested in the studies did not necessarily evaluate the minimum intake that could maintain N equilibrium.

In the study of Kountz et al. (151) three levels of protein were tested. The results of their experiments are summarized graphically in Fig. 8. From these data it was concluded that the minimum physiological requirement was 0.7 g protein/kg/day for elderly men. Since a mixed protein diet was used in the study, the data suggest that the minimum protein need of elderly men is not higher than allowances for young adult men (9). However, a body weight loss was experienced by three of the four subjects who participated in the Kountz study and it is uncertain whether the experimental diet was fully adequate for the critical assessment of minimum protein needs.

We have recently explored further the minimum protein needs of elderly women by means of the N balance approach. Our initial objective was to determine whether the 1973 FAO/WHO safe practical allowance for protein in adults was also sufficient to maintain N equilibrium in the healthy aged individual. Preliminary results from this study are summarized in Table 11 and show that, within a 28-day experimental period, most healthy people achieve N equilibrium at levels of protein intake currently considered adequate for young men and women. However, we do not know whether the minimum physiological requirement for most elderly people would be much below these levels. These preliminary findings support the views of Watkin (147) and Horwitt (150) that the minimum protein needs of healthy adults do not increase with advancing years. Furthermore, on the basis of current knowledge, the recommended intakes for healthy adults as proposed by the 1973 FAO/WHO Expert Group (9) and stated in the

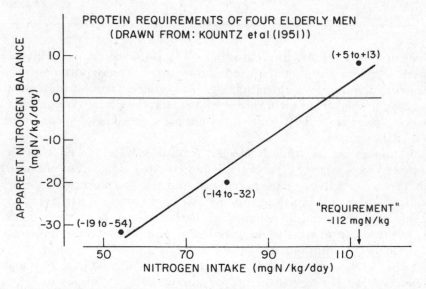

Figure 8. Relationship between apparent N balance and dietary protein intake in four men, 69–76 years old. These data were calculated from the results of Kountz et al. (151). Protein intake was provided by a mixed diet.

Table 11   Nitrogen Balance in Elderly People Given Egg Protein to Provide the 1973 FAO/WHO Safe Practical Allowance for Adult Subjects

Subject	Sex	Age (years)	Energy (Kcal/kg/day)	Protein (g/kg/day)	1 week[b]	2 weeks	4 weeks
						N Balance (g/day)[a] after	
CG	F	85	32	0.52	+0.28	+0.0	−0.5
MS	F	91	36	0.52	+0.50		
ED	F	69	38	0.52	+0.27	+0.10	
LI	F	67	33	0.52	+0.10	+1.01	
AT	F	70	28	0.52	−0.13	+0.59	
AB	F	78	31	0.52	−0.65	+0.18	
MK	F	73	34	0.52	+1.20	+0.60	+0.87
KM	F	84	33	0.52	−0.50	−0.73	−0.24
PM	M	68	36	0.57	−0.98	+0.12	+0.44
PB	M	71	24	0.57	−1.69	−1.98	−1.65

[a] Estimated "true" balance, allowing 5 mg N/kg/day for integumental and other unmeasured losses.
[b] The first week for subjects LI, AT, AB was immediately preceded by approximately a 1-week period of a free-choice diet that itself followed low-protein and protein-free diet periods.

recent edition of United States Recommended Dietary Allowances (6) appear to be adequate for most healthy elderly individuals.

EFFECTS OF INFECTION AND OTHER STRESSFUL STIMULI ON PROTEIN NEEDS

In assessing the practical and health significance of the foregoing estimates of the protein needs of individuals it is important to emphasize that the results of our own studies and the estimations for protein allowances in the elderly, as well as for young adults, are intended to apply to healthy individuals. Superimposed infection, altered gastrointestinal function, and metabolic changes which often accompany chronic disease states would all be expected to reduce the efficiency of dietary N utilization. The net result would be to increase the amount of protein needed to maintain protein nutritional status. Because elderly people are more commonly affected by these factors it is important to review, in brief, their effects on protein metabolism and nutrition. Furthermore, as Watkin (147) has stated: "Socioeconomic factors and presence of disease have far more practical influence than age per se in determining the status of protein nutrition in the aged."

The qualitative effects of acute infection on dietary protein utilization and requirements have been well described for some infections in a limited number of individuals (153). Unfortunately the available data are of little value for quantifying the effects of infection on nutrient needs in the elderly. However, it is known that infection and other stressful stimuli of physical and psychological origin produce a tendency to negative nitrogen balance through the cumulative effect of several different mechanisms.

The metabolic response to acute infection in healthy young men has been characterized by Beisel and his collaborators (154, 155). It was especially well done in a series of studies involving different types of intracellular infections, and the pattern of the metabolic response was found to be similar regardless of whether the infectious agent was a bacterium, a rickettsia, or a virus. Furthermore, nitrogen is only one of several nutrients for which there was a net body loss under such conditions because increases in the loss of potassium, magnesium, and phosphorus have been demonstrated (155) and there are changes in zinc metabolism (156).

In addition to the catabolic response of body N metabolism to infection there is a corresponding anabolic component that is of major importance during recovery from infection. Anabolic responses occur not only during recovery but also in the early phase of illness when anabolism is associated with increased production of phagocytes and other leucocytes and the induction of several tissue enzymes and of several immunoglobulins. Over-all liver protein synthesis is increased (157, 158) and skeletal muscle protein synthesis is decreased (159, 160) in response to an infectious episode.

During recovery from infection two characteristics of the anabolic period that follows are: the increased N retention seen during this period is greater than that measured during the preincubation phase, and its duration is much longer than the catabolic period (161). This may be due, in part, to the effect of protein depletion antedating the acute episode.

Digestive capacity and gastrointestinal function may also be affected by advancing age. Impaired protein digestion and fat malabsorption have been reported in older adults (162) although the mechanisms of reduced digestive capacity are not yet clear. However, it might be anticipated that a reduced ability to digest protein would lead to an increase in the amount of protein needed to maintain adequate nutritional status. In this same context, additional practical problems involve the size and distribution of meals. The distribution of nutrient intake during the day may be of considerable importance for the well-being of many elderly.

In spite of the potential for disease states to increase protein and amino acid needs in a majority of elderly people there are no studies which help to assess the quantitative influence of disease on nutrient utilization and dietary requirements. Although a complex problem (163), there is an urgent need to explore and to define the nutritional and dietary significance of disease states which are common to so many members of the elderly population.

SUMMARY AND PRACTICAL CONCLUSIONS

In this chapter we have considered some aspects of the metabolic basis for the total protein and essential amino acid needs of elderly subjects. Body protein mass declines progressively with age in human subjects and this alone should lead to a reduced need for dietary protein. There is also a fall in the rate of total body protein synthesis per unit of body weight, and a redistribution in total body protein synthesis with the metabolically active visceral organs making a more important contribution to total body N metabolism as the adult years advance. From preliminary data on the urinary excretion of 3-methylhistidine, assumed to come mainly from skeletal muscle, it appears that the rate of muscle protein synthesis is reduced with increased age and this may account for the finding, in a limited number of subjects, that the over-all rate of total body protein synthesis per unit of body cell mass is similar in young adults and aged people of the same sex and the use of essentially identical experimental techniques are needed before the relationships between dynamic measures of whole body protein metabolism and dietary protein requirements can be defined in precise, predictive terms.

Nitrogen balance studies on the estimation of needs of individual essential amino acids are limited and contradictory. A difficulty that arises in the comparative evaluation of the essential amino acid requirements of young and older subjects is that the relatively brief experimental diet periods which have been used for this purpose have not been considered for their metabolic equivalence in differing age groups. Data for threonine and tryptophan suggest that the requirements for these amino acids are similar to those for young adults, when expressed per unit of body weight, but may be higher per unit of body cell mass. An extension and confirmation of these findings is required before definitive conclusions may be drawn for the essential amino acid needs of older people.

New data on obligatory urine and fecal N losses in healthy elderly women are described and compared with published data for young men and women. Total obligatory N losses, per unit of body weight, are less for elderly women than for young men but similar to published data from earlier studies with young women. From these data, a protein allowance of 0.42 g/kg/day for elderly women is predicted by the factorial method. This estimate is identical to the value of 0.41 g/kg/day derived from the studies of Bricker and Smith (142) with young college women but lower than the 1973 FAO/WHO estimates for the "safe practical" allowance for protein in both adult men and women, which were 0.57 and 0.52 g/kg/day, respectively. Our recent studies also show that these latter allowances are sufficient to achieve body N equilibrium in most healthy elderly subjects during short-term metabolic balance periods.

The effects of infectious disease, and possible decreased digestive capacity as well as metabolic abnormalities, which affect many members of the elderly population, on dietary protein and essential amino acid requirements have been qualitatively demonstrated, but their quantitative significance requires urgent and careful evaluation. Furthermore, it is also not known whether a "safe practical" allowance is sufficient to support body N repletion and a return to metabolic normality following stressful stimuli or whether it is adequate to maintain maximum resistance to disease. Finally, the protein and amino acid needs of adult man have been based almost entirely on the metabolic N balance approach. The adequacy of this approach has not been carefully studied and there is a need for the development of new and functional approaches for determining nutrient requirements. Until these important problems are resolved through additional research, the practical significance of the "minimum physiological requirement" for protein and individual essential amino acids and the estimates for "recommended" or "safe practical" allowances derived from these data will remain highly uncertain.

ACKNOWLEDGMENT

We thank the members of our research group at Massachusetts Institute of Technology for their dedicated help during the conduct of these studies. Also, we greatly appreciate the cooperation of the subjects, both young and old, who volunteered to undertake the demands of the experimental protocols.

REFERENCES

1. Comfort, A. *Mech. Age Develop.* **3**:1 (1974).
2. Taeuber, C. *Science.* **176**:773 (1972).
3. Cohen, C. *Scot. Med. J.* **10**:42 (1965).
4. Shock, N. *J. Am. Diet. Assoc.* **56**:491 (1970).
5. Strelher, B. L. *Time, Cells and Aging.* Academic, New York, 1962.
6. National Research Council, Food & Nutrition Board. *Recommended Dietary Allowances.* 8th Revised Edition. National Academy Sciences, Washington, D.C., 1974.
7. FAO/WHO, *Requirements of Vitamin A, thiamine, riboflavin and niacin.* WHO Tech. Rept. Ser. No. 362, World Health Org., Geneva, Switzerland, 1967.
8. FAO/WHO, *Requirements of Ascorbic acid, Vitamin D, Vitamin B12, folate and iron.* FAO Nutr. Meetings Rept. Ser. No. 27, Food and Agriculture Organization, Rome, Italy, 1970.
9. FAO/WHO, *Protein and Energy Requirements.* WHO Report Ser. No. 522, World Health Organization, Geneva, Switzerland, 1973.
10. Medvedev, Zh. A. In *Advances in Gerontological Research, Vol. 1.* B. L. Strehler, Ed., Academic, New York, 1964, p. 181
11. von Hahn, H. P. In *Advances in Gerontological Research,* Vol. 3. B. L. Strehler, Ed., Academic, New York, 1971, p. 1.
12. Adelman, R. C. In *Advances in Gerontological Research,* Vol. 4. B. L. Strehler, Ed., Academic, New York, 1972, p. 1.
13. Scrimshaw, N. S., Hussein, M. A., Murray, E., Rand, W. M., and Young, V. R. *J. Nutr.* **102**:1595 (1972).
14. Cohen, S. H. and Dombrowski, C. S. *J. Nuclear Med.* **12**:499 (1971).
15. Harvey, T. C., Dykes, P. W., Chen, N. S., Ettinger, K. V., Jain, S., James, H., Chettle, D. R., Fremlin, J. H., and Thomas, B. J. *Lancet* **2**:395 (1973).
16. Cohen, S. H., Cinque, T. J., Dombrowski, C. S., and Letteri, J. M. *J. Lab. Clin. Med.* **79**:978 (1972).
17. J. Brozek and A. Henschel, Eds. *Techniques for Measuring Body Composition.* National Academy of Sciences — National Research Council, Washington, D. C. 1961.
18. Moore, F. D., Olesen, K. H., McMurrey, J. D., Parker, H. V., Ball, M. R., and Boyde, C. M. *The Body Cell Mass and its Supporting Environment.* Saunders, Philadelphia, 1963.
19. National Academy of Sciences, *Body Composition in Animals and Man.* Publication No. 1598, National Academy Sciences, Washington, D. C., 1968.
20. Allen, T. H., Anderson, E. C., and Langham, W. H. *J. Gerontol.* **15**:348 (1960).
21. Myhre, L. B. and Kessler, W. *J. Appl. Physiol.* **21**:1251 (1966).
22. Forbes, G. B. and Reina, J. C. *Metabolism* **19**:653 (1970).
23. Lesser, G. T., Kumar, I., and Steele, J. M. *Ann. N. Y. Acad. Sci.* **110**:578 (1963).

24. Nathan, D. G., Piomelli, S., Cummins, J. F., Gardner, F. H., and Limauro, A. L. *Ann. N. Y. Acad. Sci.* **110:**965 (1963).

25. Widdowson, E. M. and Dickerson, J. W. T. In *Mineral Metabolism,* Vol. 2. C. L. Comar and F. Bronner Eds. Academic, New York, 1964, part A, p. 2.

26. Forbes, G. B. and Lewis, A. M. *J. Clin. Invest.* **35:**596 (1956).

27. Andrew, W., Shock, N. W., Barrows, C. H., and Yiengst, H. J. *J. Gerontol.* **14:**405 (1959).

28. Yiengst, M. J., Barrows, C. H., and Shock, N. W. *J. Gerontol.* **14:**400 (1959).

29. Neumaster, T. D. and Ring, G. C., *J. Gerontol.* **20:**379 (1965).

30. Forbes, G. B. *Growth* **36:**325 (1972).

31. Cheek, D. B., Brasel, J. A., and Graystone, J. E. In *Human Growth.* D. B. Cheek, Ed., Lea & Febiger, Philadelphia, 1968, Chapter 22.

32. E. Jokl, Ed., *Nutrition, Exercise and Body Composition.* Thomas, Springfield, Ill., 1964.

33. Yan, S. H. Y. and Franks, J. J. *J. Lab. Clin. Med.* **72:**449 (1968).

34. Beauchene, R. E., Roeder, L. M., and Barrows, C. H. *J. Gerontol.* **22:**318 (1967).

35. Beauchene, R. E., Roeder, L. M., and Barrows, C. H. *J. Gerontol.* **25:**359 (1970).

36. Berg, B. N. *Proc. Soc. Exp. Biol. Med.* **119:**417 (1965).

37. Everitt, A. V. *Gerontologia* **2:**33 (1958).

38. Sanadi, D. R. and Fletcher, M. J. In *Biological Aspects of Aging.* N. W. Shock, Ed., New York, Columbia Univ. Press, 1962, p. 298.

39. Menzies, R. A. and Gold, P. H. *J. Biol. Chem.* **246:**2425 (1971).

40. Chen J. C., Ove, P., and Lansing, A. J. *Biochem. Biophys. Acta.* **312:**598 (1973).

41. Hrachovec, J. P. *Gerontologia* **17:**75.

42. Mainwaring, M. I. P. *Biochem. J.* **113:**869 (1969).

43. Young, V. R. In *Mammalian Protein Metabolism,* Vol. IV. H. N. Munro, Ed., Academic, New York, 1970, Chapter 40.

44. Young, V. R. *J. Anim. Sci.* **38:**1054 (1974).

45. Breuer, C. B. and Florini, J. R. *Biochemistry* **4:**1544 (1965).

46. Srivastava U. and Chaudhary, K. D. *Can. J. Biochem.* **47:**231 (1969).

47. Srivastava, U. *Arch. Biochem. Biophys.* **130:**129 (1969).

48. Lerner, M. P. and Johnson, T. C. *J. Biol. Chem.* **245:**1388 (1970).

49. Munro, H. N. and Gray, J. A. M. *Comp. Biochem Physiol.* **28:**897 (1969).

50. Miller, S. A. In *Mammalian Protein Metabolism,* Vol. III. H. N. Munro, Ed., Academic, New York, 1969, Chapter 26.

51. Pawlak, M. and Pion, R. *Ann. Biol. Anim. Biochem. Biophys.* **8:**517 (1968).

52. Elwyn, D. H. In *Mammalian Protein Metabolism,* Vol. IV. H. N. Munro, Ed., Academic, New York, 1970, Chapter 38.

53. Peraino, C. and Harper, A. E. *J. Nutr.* **80:**270 (1963).

54. Wehr, R. F. and Lewis, G. T. *Proc. Soc. Exp. Biol. Med.* **121:**349 (1966).

55. Armstrong, M. D. and Stave, U. *Metabolism* **22:**571 (1973).

56. Theimer, V. W. *Naturwissenschafun* **51:**465 (1964).

57. Young V. R. and Scrimshaw N. S. In *Protein and Amino Acid Functions,* Vol. II. E. J. Bigwood, Ed., Pogamar, New York, 1972, p. 541.

58. Waterlow, J. C. and Stephen, J. M. L. *Clin. Sci.* **33**:489 (1967).

59. Waterlow, J. C. and Stephen, J. M. L. *Clin. Sci.* **35**:287 (1968).

60. Yousef, M. K. and Johnson, H. D. *Proc. Soc. Exp. Biol. Med.* **133**:1351 (1970).

61. Waterlow, J. C. *Nutr. Revs.* **28**:115 (1970).

62. Picou, D. and Taylor-Roberts, T. *Clin. Sci.* **36**:283 (1969).

63. Waterlow, J. C. In *Mammalian Protein Metabolism,* Vol. III. H. N. Munro, Ed., Academic, New York, 1970, Chapter 28.

64. Sharp, C. S., Larsen, S., Shankman, S., Hazlet, J. W. and Kednis, M. S. *J. Nutr.* **63**:155 (1957).

65. Shipley, R. A. and Clark, R. E. *Tracer Methods for in vivo Kinetics,* Academic, New York, 1972.

66. Muldowney, F. P., Crooks, J. and Bluhm, M. M. *J. Clin. Invest.* **36**:1375 (1957).

67. Alleyne, G. A. O., Viteri, F. and Alvarado, J. *Am. J. Clin. Nutr.* **23**:875 (1970).

68. Graystone, J. E. In *Human Growth.* D. B. Cheek, Ed., Lea & Febiger, Philadelphia, 1968, p. 182.

69. Bertolini, A. M. *Gerontologic Metabolism,* C. C. Thomas, Springfield, Ill. 1969, p. 660.

70. Haverberg, L. N., Munro, H. N. and Young, V. R. *Biochem. Biophys. Acta.* (in press).

71. Young, V. R., Alexis, S. D., Baliga, B. S., Munro, H. N. and Muecke, W. *J. Biol. Chem.* **247**:3592 (1972).

72. Long, C. H., Haverberg, L. N., Kinney, J. M., Young, V. R., Munro, H. N. and Geiger, J. W. *Metabolism* (in press).

73. Long, C. L., Young, V. R., Kinney, J. M., Munro, H. N., Haverberg, L. N. and Geiger, J. W. *Fed. Proc.* **33**:691 (Abstr.) (1974).

74. Young, V. R., Haverberg, L. N., Bilmazes, C. and Munro, H. N. *Metabolism* **22**:1429 (1973).

75. Asatoor, A. M. and Armstrong, M. D. *Biochem Biophys. Res. Comm.* **26**:168 (1967).

76. Henshaw, E. C., Hirsch, C. A., Milosevic, P. and Hiatt, H. H. *Trans. Assoc. Am. Physicians* **81**:116 (1968).

77. Gan, J. C. and Jeffay, H. *Biochem. Biophys. Acta.* **148**:448 (1967).

78. Watkin, D. M. In *Mammalian Protein Metabolism,* Vol. II. H. N. Munro and J. B. Alleson, Eds., Academic, New York, 1964, Chapter 17.

79. Watkin, D. M. In *World Review of Nutrition & Dietetics,* Vol. 6. G. H. Bourne, Ed., S. Karger, Basel/New York, 1966, p. 124.

80. Munro, H. N. In *Nutrition in Old Age,* L. A. Carlson, Ed., Swedish Nutrition Foundation, Uppsala, Sweden, 1972, p. 32.

81. Irwin, M. and Hegsted, D. M. *J. Nutr.* **101**:539 (1971).

82. Nagakawa, I., Takahashi, T., Suzuki, T. and Kobayaski, K. *J. Nutr.* **80**:305 (1964).

83. Rose, W. C. *Nutr. Abstr. Revs.* **27**:631 (1957).

84. Holt, L. E. and Snyderman, S. E. *Nutr. Abstr. Revs.* **35**:1 (1965).

85. Leverton, R. M., Gram, M. R., Chaloupka, M., Brodovsky, E. and Mitchell, A. *J. Nutr.* **58**:59 (1956).

86. Tuttle, S. G., Swendseid, M. E., Mulcare, D., Griffith, W. H. and Bassett, S. H. *Metabolism* **6**:564 (1957).

87. Tuttle, S. G., Swendseid, M. E., Mulcare, D., Griffith, W. H. and Bassett, S. H. *Metabolism* **8:**61 (1959).

88. Tuttle, S. G., Bassett, S. H., Griffith, W. H., Mulcare, D. B. and Swendseid, M. E. *Am. J. Clin. Nutr.* **16:**225 (1965).

89. Tuttle, S. G., Bassett, S. H., Griffith, W. H., Mulcare, D. B. and Swendseid, M. E. *Am. J. Clin. Nutr.* **16:**229 (1965).

90. Watts, J. H., Mann, A. N., Bradley, L. and Thompson, D. J. *J. Gerontol.* **19:**370 (1964).

91. FAO/WHO, *Protein Requirements.* WHO Tech. Rept. Ser. No. 301, World Health Organization, Geneva, Switzerland, 1965.

92. Gaull, G., Sturman, J. A. and Räihä, N.C.R. *Pediat. Res.* **6:**538 (1972).

93. Munro, H. N. In *Mammalian Protein Metabolism,* Vol. IV. H. N. Munro, Ed., Academic, New York, 1970, p. 340.

94. McLaughlan, J. M. and Morrison, A. B. In *Protein Nutrition and Free Amino Acid Patterns* J. H. Leathem, Ed., Rutgers Univ. Press, New Brunswick, N. J., 1968, pp. 3–18.

95. Richardson, L. R., Blaylock, L. G. and Lyman, C. M. *J. Nutr.* **49:**21 (1953).

96. Hill, D. C. and Olsen, E. M. *J. Nutr.* **79:**303 (1963).

97. Young, V. R. and Zamora J. *J. Nutr.* **96:**21 (1968).

98. Swendseid, M. E., Villalobos, J. and Fredrich, B. *J. Nutr.* **80:**99 (1963).

99. Puchal, F., Hays, V. W., Speer, V. C., Jones, J. D. and Catron, D. V. *J. Nutr.* **76:**11 (1963).

100. Longnecker, J. B. and Hause, N. L. *Am. J. Clin. Nutr.* **4:**356 (1961).

101. Swendseid, M. E., Tuttle, S. G., Gigueroa, W. S., Mulcare, D., Clark, A. J. and Massey, F. J. *J. Nutr.* **88:**239 (1966).

102. Snyderman, S. E., Boyer, A., Norton, P. M., Roitman, E. and Holt, L. E., Jr. *Am. J. Clin. Nutr.* **15:**313 (1964).

103. Longnecker, J. B. and Hause, N. L. *Arch. Biochem. Biophys.* **84:**46 (1959).

104. Dean, W. F. and Scott, H. M. *J. Nutr.* **88:**75 (1966).

105. Smith, R. E. and Scott, H. M. *J. Nutr.* **86:**45 (1965).

106. Zimmerman, R. A. and Scott, H. M. *J. Nutr.* **87:**13 (1965).

107. Pawlak, M. and Pion, R. *Ann. Biol. Anim. Biochem. Biophys.* **8:**517 (1968).

108. Stockland, W.L., Meade, R. J., and Melliere, A. L. *J. Nutr.* **100:**925 (1970).

109. McLaughlan, J. M. and Illman, W. I. *J. Nutr.* **93:**21 (1967).

110. R. Kihlberg, *Evaluation of Novel Protein Products* In *Proceedings of the International Biological Programme and Wenner-Gren Center Symposium.* A. E. Bender, B. Lofqvist and L. Munck, Eds., 1970, p. 149

111. Mitchell, J. R., Becker, D. E., Jensen, A. H., Harmon, B. G., and Norton, H. W. *J. Anim. Sci.* **27:**1327 (1968).

112. Bravo, F. O., Meade, J., Stockland, W. L. and Nordstrom, J. W. *J. Anim. Sci.* **31:**1137 (1970).

113. Nimrick, K. Hatfield, E. E., Kaminski, J., and Owens, F. N. *J. Nutr.* **100:**1301 (1970).

114. Young, V. R., Hussein, M. A., Murray, E., and Scrimshaw, N. S. *J. Nutr.* **101:**45 (1971).

115. Young, V. R., Tontisirin, K., Ozalp, J., Lakshmanan, F. and Scrimshaw, N. S. *J. Nutr.* **102:**1159 (1972).

116. Tontisirin, K., Young, V. R., Rand, W. M., and Scrimshaw, N. S. *J. Nutr.***104:**495 (1974).

117. Tontisirin, K., Young, V. R., and Scrimshaw, N. S. *J. Nutr.* **25:**976 (1972).

118. Tontisirin, K., Young, V. R., Miller, M., and Scrimshaw, N. S. *J. Nutr.* **103:**1220 (1973).

119. Weller, L. A., Calloway, D. H., Margen, S. *J. Nutr.* **101:**1499 (1971).

120. H. E. Clark, In *Newer Methods of Nutritional Biochemistry,* Vol. II. A. A. Albanese, Ed., Academic, New York, 1965, Chapter 4.

121   Swendseid, M. E., Watts, J. H., Harris, C. L. and Tuttle, S. G. *J. Nutr.* **75:**295 (1961).

122. Swendseid, M. E., Harris, C. L., and Tuttle, S. G. *J. Nutr.* **77:**391 (1962).

123. Leverton, R. M. and Steel, D. *J. Nutr.* **78:**10 (1962).

124. Watts, J. H., Tolbert, B., and Ruff, N. L. *Can. J. Biochem. and Physiol.* **42:**1437 (1964).

125. Kirk, M. C., Metheny, N., and Reynolds, M. S. *J. Nutr.* **77:**448 (1962).

126. Kolski, S. M., Shannon, B., Howe, J. M., and Clark, H. E. *Am. J. Clin. Nutr.* **22:**21 (1969).

127. Clark, H. E., Myers, P., Goyal, K., and Rinehart, J. *Am. J. Clin. Nutr.* **18:**91 (1966).

128. Scrimshaw, N. S., Bressani, R., Behar, M., and Viteri, F. *J. Nutr.* **66:**485 (1958).

129. Krishnaswamy, K. and Gopalan, C. *Lancet* **2:**1167 (1971).

130. Sugahara, M., Baker, D. H., and Scott, H. M. *J. Nutr.* **97:**29 (1969).

131. Swendseid, M. E., Harris, C. L., and Tuttle, S. G. *J. Nutr.* **71:**105 (1960).

132. Kies, C. and Fox, H. M. *J. Nutr.* **100:**1275 (1970).

133. Kies, C. F., Shortridge, L., and Reynolds, M. S. *J. Nutr.* **85:**260 (1965).

134. Irwin, M. I. and Hegsted, D. M. *J. Nutr.* **101:**385 (1971).

135. Sirbu, E. R., Margen, S., and Calloway, D. H. *Am. J. Clin. Nutr.* **20:**1158 (1967).

136. Calloway, D. H., Odell, A. C. F., and Margen, S. *J. Nutr.* **101:**775 (1971).

137. Kraut, H. and Müller-Wecker, *Hoppe-Seyler's Z. Physiol. Chem.* **320:**241 (1960).

138. Calloway, D. H. and Margen, S. *J. Nutr.* **101:**205 (1971).

139. Young, V. R., Taylor, Y. S. M., Rand, W. M., and Scrimshaw, N. S. *J. Nutr.* **103:**1164 (1973).

140. Inoue, G., Fujita, Y., and Niiyama, Y. *J. Nutr.* **103:**1673 (1973).

141. Chan, H. and Waterlow, J. C. *Brit. J. Nutr.* **20:**775 (1966).

142. Bricker, M. and Smith, J. *J. Nutr.***44:**553 (1951).

143. Forbes, G. B. *Am. J. Clin. Nutr.* **27:**595 (1974).

144. Young, V. R. and Scrimshaw, N. S. *Brit. J. Nutr.* **22:**9 (1968).

145. Hawley, E. E., Murlin, J. R., Nassett, E. S., and Szymanski, T. A. *J. Nutr.* **36:**153 (1946).

146. Murlin, J. R., Edwards, L. E., Hawley, E. E., and Clark, L. C. *J. Nutr.* **31:**533 (1946).

147. Watkin, D. M. *Ann. New York Acad. Sci.* **69:**102 (1957-58).

148. Roberts, P. H., Kerr, C. H., and Ohlson, M. A. *J. Am. Diet. Assoc.* **24:**292 (1948).

149. Albanese, A. A., Higgons, R. A., Orto, L . A., and Zwattoro, D. N. *Geriatrics* **12:**465 (1957).

150. Horwitt, M. K. *J. Am. Diet. Assoc.* **29:**443 (1953).

151. Kountz, W. B., Hofstatter, B. L., and Ackermann, P. G. *J. Gerontol.* **6:**20 (1951).

152. Albanese, A. A., Higgons, R. A., Vestal, B., Stephanson, L., and Malsch, M. *Geriatrics* **7:**109 (1952).

153. Scrimshaw, N. S., Taylor, C. E., and Gordon, J. E. *Interactions of Nutrition and Injestion,* Monograph Series No. 57, World Health Organization, Geneva, Switzerland, 1968.

154. Beisel, W. R. *Fed. Proc.* **25:**1682 (1966).

155. Beisel, W. R., Sawyer, W. D., Ryll, E. D. and Crozier, D. *Am. Intern. Med.* **67:**744 (1967).

156. Powanda, M. C., Cockerell, G. L., and Pekarek, R. S. *Am. J. Physiol.* **225:**399 (1973).

157   Lust, G. *Fed. Proc.* **25:**1688 (1966).

158. Symons, L. E. A., Jones, W. D., and Steel, J. W. *Exp. Parasitol.* **35:**492 (1974).

159. Young, V. R., Chen, S. C., and Newberne, P. M. *J. Nutr.* **94:**361 (1968).

160. Symons, L. E. A. and Jones, W. D. *Exp. Parasitol.* **29:**230 (1971).

161. Beisel, W. R. *Am. J. Clin. Nutr.* **25:**1254 (1972).

162. Werner, J. and Hambracus, L. In *Nutrition in Old Age* L. A. Carlson, Ed., Swedish Nutrition Foundation, Uppsala, Sweden, 1972, p. 55.

163. Levenson, S. M. and Watkin, D. M. *Fed. Proc.* **18:**1155 (1959).

6

Life Style and Nutrient Intake
in the Elderly

E. NEIGE TODHUNTER, Ph.D.

Biochemistry Department, Vanderbilt University Medical School, Nashville, Tennessee

A major factor in enabling the elderly to continue independent living is their ability to obtain or prepare meals adequate to maintain their nutritional health. Comparatively few studies have been made to determine the adequacy of the diets of older age groups. There have been some at the local and others at the national levels (USDA Household Consumption Survey, 1965; Ten State Survey; and "HANES"). Still fewer investigations have attempted to determine the factors that contribute to dietary inadequacy by looking more closely at the life styles.

The investigation partially reported here* was undertaken to identify factors that influence the food practices, acceptance, and attitudes of elderly persons, and to determine the extent to which group-feeding programs are needed, and should be modified, according to region, socioeconomic status, ethnicity, sex, and other possible factors.

This investigation was made during February to December, 1973. These dates are important because of the marked increase in food prices since that time, and some findings reported here might be different if the same study were repeated today.

---

*"Food Acceptance and Food Attitudes of the Elderly as a Basis for Planning Nutrition Programs." E. Neige Todhunter, Faye House, Roger Vander Zwaag (Vanderbilt University). Tennessee Commission on Aging, Nashville, Tenn. June, 1974. p. 178.

THE SAMPLE AND METHODS USED

The sample of individuals 60 years and over of noninstitutionalized persons in middle Tennessee included both males and females, and blacks and whites, with different educational levels, socioeconomic backgrounds, and living conditions, from both rural and urban areas, who were willing and competent to be interviewed. The total group of 529 persons interviewed had a mean age of 73.6 years, median 72.3 years, mode 75 years, and a range of 60 to 102 years (Table 1).

Table 1   Characteristics of the Sample

Characteristic	Total Number	Male	Female	Black	White	Rural	Urban
Age[a]							
60-64	65	27	38	14	51	20	45
65-69	105	34	71	30	75	26	79
70-74	121	39	82	52	69	17	104
75-79	117	42	75	36	81	18	99
80-84	71	20	51	22	49	13	58
over 85	49	23	26	19	30	6	43
Education							
none	10	9	1	7	3	2	8
grades	279	106	173	135	144	51	228
high school	145	44	101	18	127	29	116
college	73	16	57	10	63	14	59
degree received	22	10	12	3	19	5	17
Marital status							
single	56	11	45	11	45	9	47
married	169	112	57	47	122	59	110
widowed[b]	304	62	242	115	189	33	271
Living							
alone	287	58	229	111	176	20	267
with spouse	167	109	55	47	117	57	107
with relatives	67	15	52	13	54	20	47
with friend	11	3	8	2	9	4	7

[a]One urban white female age not given.
[b]Includes also divorced or separated.

All data were obtained by personal interview and all interviews were by the same qualified dietitian, familiar with regional terminology and food practices, skilled in establishing rapport, and experienced in working with the elderly. The interview was limited to questions that could be answered in about 60 minutes, and thus could be completed without tiring the respondent. A 24-hour food recall was obtained and intake of seven nutrients was calculated.

DATA TREATMENT

For a few questions where the replies varied with the individuals a hand count was made. All other data were keypunched on cards and computer analyses were made. All data are presented as percentages of the total group or of subgroups (race and sex). Averages have not been used because we believe this tends to obscure major differences within the groups or between groups.

DESCRIPTION OF THE SAMPLE

Living Conditions

More than half the total group (54%) lived alone, either because they were single (11%) or because they were widowed, divorced, or separated. The highest percentage of single individuals was among white women.

Two-thirds of the group were renters, and 44% lived in apartments. All participants had food preparation and food storage facilities; electricity was used by 95%. Approximately three-fourths of each subgroup made food purchases at supermarkets and the remainder mainly at neighborhood stores. About 40% shopped once a week and 36% from two to four times per week. Black women shopped least frequently, probably because of transportation problems and distance from food markets (3 miles for half of this subgroup). The majority of each subgroup were within one-half mile of markets and public transportation systems.

Financial Status

No direct question regarding amount of income was asked but from information available about sources of income and rent, it was possible to make a reliable estimate of income. Twenty-nine percent of the total group had an individual income below $1800, 20% between $1800 and $2400, 28% between $2400 and $5000, and 22% over $5000. More blacks were in the lowest income group.

Money spent for food was $5.00 or less per week by 9% (mainly blacks) and between $5.00 and $10.00 by 48%, and 24 percent spent $10 to $15 per week.

Aloneness

Aloneness was considered because of the possible effect on food practices. To live alone does not necessarily mean loneliness, which is largely dependent on the interests and inner resources of the individual. A high proportion lived alone, but only 7% of the total group never had any visits with relatives (and this was about the same by race and sex). Daily visits with relatives were the normal occurrence for 44% of the total group, with males having the highest percentage and black women the lowest (25%). Religious affiliation was high for both sexes and races and there was church attendance by 69% of the total group, with the highest percentage being the black female group (76%).

About 13% of the total group did not participate in recreational activities of any kind, and 22% of the black women had no recreation. The highest percentage of each subgroup engaged in recreation that did not involve others (such as walking, gardening, sewing, fishing, reading, and music listening).

Volunteer services in the community were participated in by 13%, more often by females than males. About 12% had some employment, either at regular hours or irregularly.

Loneliness did not seem to be a major problem for this group; however, no information was obtained on their inner feelings.

Those who lived alone and those who lived with others (spouse, relatives, or friends) when compared as subgroups did *not* differ in dietary adequacy.

Health Status

The health of individuals may influence their current food practices. Health of participants in this study was evaluated from their responses to the interviewer regarding how they felt physically, what they thought their ailments were, what their physician had told them, their dental condition, their use of prescribed medication and vitamin or mineral supplements, and their mobility and physical ability to prepare food.

More than 50% of males, both black and white, claimed to feel healthy, but only 30% of the black and the white females answered affirmatively. Incidence of arthritis was higher among women (30%) than men (13%). None of the black men expressed a desire to lose weight; 10% of the black women considered themselves overweight. Eighty-four percent of all participants said they had normal mobility.

Based on reports by participants of their physicians' diagnoses, a higher percentage of black women reported diabetes, heart disease, hypertension, and arthritis than any other subgroup. More black men and women reported hypertension than the white group. Sixty percent of the total group said they "feel good"; fewer white women gave this response than any other subgroup. More white women than any other subgroup took medication, and also used vitamin and mineral supplements (22%).

Ten percent of the total group were edentulous, and 16% of the group said they had chewing problems.

These health factors might be expected to affect the food practices, but this was not apparent in the dietary ratings of the groups.

FOOD PRACTICES AND BELIEFS

The Recommended Dietary Allowances (RDA), 1974, of the National Research Council are not requirements; they are allowances intended for use in planning group meals. They cannot be used for judging dietary adequacy for individuals. They were used in this study as a basis of comparison of individuals when grouped by race, sex, age, income, education, and health factors. The percentage in each group whose individual calculated nutrient intakes were 66% or more of the RDA have been classified as "satisfactory."

Nutrient Intakes

Intakes for seven essential nutrients are shown in Table 2.

Protein

More than 80% of males, both black and white, and white females, had "satisfactory" ratings, but only 70% of the black females achieved this rating. One-half of the total group met or exceeded the RDA, but only one-third of the black females met the RDA for protein.

Calcium

Two-thirds the total group had "satisfactory" ratings; fewer black females had this rating.

Table 2   Percent by Sex, Race, Age, Education, and Income with Dietary Rating of Satisfactory or Better for Seven Nutrients

Sample Descriptor	Protein %	Cal-cium %	Iron %	Vitamin A %	Thi-amin %	Ribo-flavin %	Vitamin C %
Race and sex							
Total group	84.6	66.7	54.9	44.1	43.0	37.0	67.1
Males, black	88.7	64.5	67.7	46.7	32.5	37.1	56.5
Males, white	91.0	69.7	77.9	45.9	59.0	37.7	65.6
Total males	90.2	67.8	74.4	46.1	51.1	37.4	62.5
Females, black	70.4	57.5	37.1	46.3	23.1	27.8	72.2
Females, white	86.7	70.1	47.9	41.5	45.7	41.1	68.4
Total females	81.5	65.9	44.3	42.8	38.5	36.8	69.5
Age Groups							
60–70 years	88.1	63.0	57.3	41.6	49.5	37.0	67.7
71–80 years	80.4	66.4	54.5	46.8	37.8	36.2	66.8
over 80 years	87.7	67.5	51.0	41.8	41.8	38.8	64.4
Education, formal							
None	70.0	50.0	30.0	20.0	10.0	20.0	50.0
Grade School	80.5	63.7	50.7	40.6	38.0	36.6	58.3
High School	88.3	66.2	60.0	48.3	46.2	32.4	75.2
College	94.6	75.3	58.9	49.3	54.7	43.8	79.8
Degree received	86.3	86.4	72.7	54.5	59.1	59.1	90.9
Income							
Low	78.8	65.4	42.3	27.9	30.8	36.5	58.7
Middle	82.8	62.4	50.7	46.6	38.9	34.4	62.9
High	89.6	72.1	66.2	49.8	53.7	40.3	76.1

Iron

There was a marked difference between the numbers of men and women in iron intakes; 78% of males (black and white) but only 48% of white females and 37% of black females met the "satisfactory" level.

Vitamin A

More than half the total group had less than "satisfactory" intakes, but over 40% of blacks (both male and female) met the RDA.

Thiamin

More than half the total groups were below "satisfactory" rating, and blacks (male and female) had the least number with this rating.

Riboflavin

Riboflavin was the nutrient of lowest intake by the total group, with little difference between races or sexes.

Vitamin C

Intakes of Vitamin C were "satisfactory" for two-thirds of the total group, with black females having the largest number with the "satisfactory" rating (72%).

Comparison of dietary ratings by age groups, between those with and without problems in chewing food, between those who did and did not "feel poorly," and between those living alone or with others showed no appreciable differences.

Dietary ratings were influenced by level of formal education and by income (Table 2), which is in agreement with findings in national and other surveys. The number of satisfactory ratings for all nutrients improved up through the group having some high school education. As income increased, more participants met the adequacy standard for all nutrients.

The above dietary data have been presented from the point of view of the percentage of each subgroup who had ratings of satisfactory or better. The problem of adequate nutrient intake is further emphasized if one studies how many individuals had diets providing less than one-third the RDA for various nutrients. In this classification it was found that one-fifth the total group had less than one-third the RDA for vitamin C, one-third the RDA for riboflavin, and one-fourth the RDA for vitamin A.

These data indicate that there are differences in the diets consumed by males and females and also differences between those of blacks and whites. More diets of blacks were satisfactory in vitamin A, and low in thiamin than for whites. More black women had diets of lower rating in protein, calcium, and iron but higher in vitamin C than any other subgroups.

Study of actual foods consumed indicated that size of servings rather than choice of foods was a major factor influencing the nutrient intake.

Beliefs about Food and Health

In response to a question about what foods are "good for health" approximately 14% of black males and females and white males said all foods were good; only 5% of white females gave this response. Vegetables were named more often than any other food by both races and sexes, and this belief was consistent with their actual practice. Foods usually considered "health foods" were not mentioned.

Pork was most frequently mentioned as "bad for health." Foods high in fat or fried foods were named by more than 10% of each subgroup and most frequently by black males (20%). Sweets (desserts and candy) also were considered in this category by about 10% of the participants.

Approximately 90% of each subgroup believed their own diet was good and that the food they ate affected the way they felt; 84% of each subgroup said they had a good appetite for meals.

The use of vitamin or mineral supplements was comparatively low. It occurred in about 15% of the white males and females and was almost negligible among blacks.

Willingness to try new foods was expressed by 60% of each subgroup. More than 50% of white males and females and 75% of black males and females, believed food had "less taste" than it used to have. Approximately 70% of each subgroup had made some changes in food habits, mostly in recent years, for reasons of health, aloneness, beliefs, and a few for financial reasons.

Companionship was considered the most important factor at mealtime by 41% of white females, 34% of white males, 27% of black males and 25% of black females. "Food you like" and the way it is cooked were rated important by 30% of white females and 36% of black females.

More than 50% of the total group had a favorable attitude to the need for food and did not economize by reducing food expenditures. More blacks than whites did economize on food. Meat was the food first to be economized on.

Breakfast was eaten regularly by over 90% of the group, was eaten at home, and was the favorite meal for more than one-third of each subgroup.

Comparatively few meals were eaten away from home and least often by black women.

Interviewees were asked to name their favorite foods and most disliked foods (no check list was given; these were spontaneous answers). Meat of some kind was mentioned most frequently (beef by 37%, chicken by 24%, and pork by 10%); next in frequency was green beans (32%), greens (25%), and potatoes (16%). Fifteen percent said they had no disliked foods. Many different foods were listed as disliked, but cottage cheese was most frequently mentioned (by 13%). Few could give any reasons for disliking a food; taste was most frequently mentioned, but dislike of some vegetables was because of their texture or because "they disagree with me."

Fresh produce was preferred by all subgroups, but canned foods were used by 85% and frozen foods less frequently by blacks.

Between-meal eating, or snacks, was the regular practice of only 37% of the total group. The kind of snack foods used were predominantly protein-rich foods or dairy products; beverages were infrequent snack choices.

SUMMARY

The life styles of the elderly population under study indicate that they had positive attitudes toward health in general and toward food and eating. Their food habits and beliefs were free from faddism, they were willing to try new foods and to change at least some of their food habits, and they had a good appetite for meals. Meal patterns and choice of foods, snacks, and food likes were toward foods of high nutritive value. They had comparatively few food dislikes, and the majority ate three meals a day.

Many of the participants in this study had nutrient intakes of less than two-thirds the 1974 RDAs. Food choices, meal patterns, and beliefs about food suggest that economic factors strongly influenced dietary adequacy and limited the food choices and size of servings. Black females appear to be the most disadvantaged group.

All of these findings are a strong indicator of the need for group feeding programs for the elderly. Such meal programs should provide at least one-third of the daily nutrient needs, and should be pleasurable experiences using foods appropriate to the food habits and beliefs of the specific groups, their locale, and their cultural-economic backgrounds. These programs should also be accompanied by realistic nutrition education programs designed to provide guidance in buying and using foods of highest nutritive value within their resources. The need for such programs becomes increasingly urgent because of today's rapidly increasing food prices.

PART 3

Nutrition-Related Diseases of Old Age

7

Prevention and Treatment of Osteoporosis

JENIFER JOWSEY, D.PHIL.

Mayo Clinic and Mayo Foundation, Rochester, Minnesota

In the past, fracture of the femoral neck frequently was a terminal illness, the cause of death being postoperative complications, commonly pneumonia. Modern techniques and the use of antibiotics have made this a rare phenomenon. However, the pain and disability caused by femoral neck and, perhaps more often, spinal fractures are encountered in considerable numbers of cases by physicians and orthopedic surgeons and thus constitute a significant medical problem. The fractures are the result of loss of bone mass to the extent that a skeleton, or a part of it, fails to support the body.

OSTEOPOROSIS

Osteoporosis with symptoms probably occurs in one-third of women over the age of 60 years and is found in both men and women of younger ages. The age at onset of the disease appears to be decreasing, and osteoporosis may well become one of the most common problems in the future.

An osteoporotic person is defined symptomatically as one with pain and disability resulting from fractures, generally a femoral neck fracture or one or more fractures of vertebrae. It has been helpful to define the disease by the degree of bone loss, using quantitative roent-

This investigation was supported in part by Research Grant AM-8658 from the National Institutes of Health, Public Health Service.

131

genologic features such as bone cortical thickness or the femoral trabecular pattern index (the Singh index) (1, 2). The Singh index is based on the disappearance of trabeculae from the neck and head region of the femur. As bone is lost, the trabecular bundles are resorbed in inverse order of the stress placed on them (Fig. 1). The

Trabecular Grading Patterns (Singh)

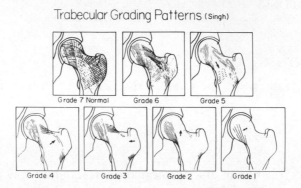

Grade 7 Normal   Grade 6   Grade 5

Grade 4   Grade 3   Grade 2   Grade I

Figure 1.   Trabecular patterns in proximal femur, showing grading according to presence or absence of major trabeculae. Arrows point to the differentiating feature.

method has the advantage of being independent of body weight and therefore differs from bone densitometry and mass measurements, which are blurred by the influence of skeletal size. In osteoporotic persons the Singh index is grade 1, 2, or 3; a person with a Singh index of grade 4 may not have symptoms, and such a value might indicate the need for preventive treatment.

Before the development of the Singh index, it was impossible to evaluate skeletal status to determine if bone mass was decreased to the point where the risk of fracture was high. This is now possible, and it would be reasonable for persons more than 45 or 50 years old to have a roentgenogram of the hip and a Singh index determination made so that preventive therapy could be instituted if indicated. Prevention of the symptoms is a far better approach than attempting to reverse the symptoms once they have occurred.

The definition of the disease remains dependent on the presence or absence of symptoms resulting from fracture. It must be remembered that a symptomatic patient with a recent fracture is expressing evidence of a long history of the process of bone loss. Also, a nonsymptomatic, and therefore "normal," person may have the same degree of bone loss as a patient with diagnosed osteoporosis, having failed to sustain a fracture only because no stress has occurred. It is obvious, therefore, that in any population there will be considerable overlap between persons with symptomatic osteoporosis and nonsymptomatic controls when bone mass, bone turnover rates, and hormonal aberrations are studied. The disease or pain reflects rate of bone loss, duration of bone loss, and recent stress. A fracture results from both a decreased amount of bone and stress; if the stress does not occur and there is no fracture, then the patient is classified as normal.

Decrease in bone mass, which is the significant feature of osteoporosis, appears to be caused by an increase in resorption of bone relative to its deposition. Morphologically, there is a decrease in the number of trabeculae in the spongy bone (Fig. 2A). Cortical bone becomes more porotic and tends to disappear on the endosteal surface (Fig. 2B). The loss of bone appears to be related to need: bone that has important weight-bearing functions tends to be protected. The outer third of the cortex of long bones and the vertically oriented trabeculae of the vertebrae and ends of the long bones remain and appear to be resistant to resorption. Clearly, bone does not disappear completely, and it has been suggested that, as osteoporosis develops, the increased stress on a decreased skeletal mass somehow prevents further loss in spite of the continued influence of the factors that resulted in the decrease of bone tissue.

When the loss of bone has decreased the skeletal mass to the level at which it fails to respond any more to hormonal influences, then the skeleton is behaving primarily as a supporting organ. Up until this point, the skeleton also is functioning as a calcium reserve. Calcium is one of the most important elements in the body, with essential functions in muscle contraction, nerve conduction, and membrane transport. For body function, maintaining a serum calcium level greater than 6.0 mg/dl is far more important than maintaining skeletal mass. Although the body supply of calcium is almost exclusively in bone, calcium can be obtained from the diet. Calcium balance for homeostasis is therefore dependent on the skeleton and on the dietary intake of calcium.

Compared with cortical bone, trabecular bone has a high surface-to-volume ratio. Because the cells responsible for bone remodeling, the osteoclasts and osteoblasts, lie on the surface of bone, trabecular bone will be significantly more responsive to changes in hormone levels or other factors that cause bone loss. Decreases in mass therefore will be more apparent in regions of bone with a high proportion of trabecular bone, because most methods for detecting changes depend on percentage loss rather than absolute loss. Such regions are found in the characteristic sites of fracture, the vertebrae and the femoral neck. However, because equally "trabecular" bones (for example, the lower

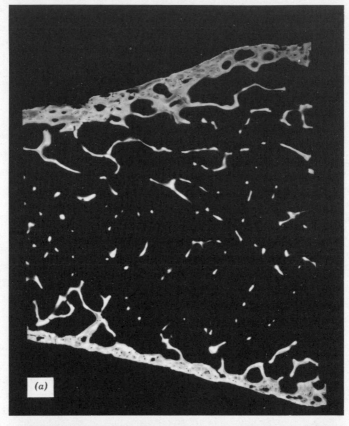

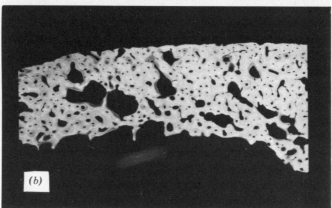

Figure 2.   Microradiographs (×8). (*A*) Iliac crest biopsy from postmenopausal osteoporotic woman. (*B*) Cross section of femur from postmenopausal osteoporotic woman.

end of the tibia) do not fracture commonly, it is apparent that stress patterns also are important and possibly are more important.

A distinction that must be made in any discussion of calcium and osteoporosis is the difference between osteoporosis and osteomalacia. If the calcium supply is deficient, then bone is resorbed to provide calcium and to maintain the serum calcium concentration within normal limits. The parathyroid glands play a major role and contain the feedback mechanism necessary to sense changes in the concentration of ionized calcium in the blood and to alter the secretion rate of the hormone accordingly. The hormone in turn causes osteoclastic bone resorption, which releases calcium and phosphate into the serum, resulting in an increase in serum calcium levels. In some instances, such as an extended period of calcium depletion or calcium lack coupled with endogenous calcium loss, a normal serum calcium level cannot be maintained; then, new bone mineralization is incomplete and osteoid remains uncalcified, resulting eventually in osteomalacia. Osteomalacia, with few exceptions, will therefore always be preceded by a period of osteoporosis. Morphologically, osteoid tissue appears on the surface of bone that is decreased in mass. Exceptions are the morphologic osteomalacia or the hyperosteoidosis of parathyroidectomy, or osteosclerotic renal osteodystrophy and endemic fluorosis.

ETIOLOGY AND TREATMENT OF OSTEOPOROSIS

For any disease, generally speaking, etiology and treatment are related. However, the etiology of osteoporosis is both multifactorial and, to some extent, unknown. Inasmuch as there are concrete data to support certain causes of the disease, it is worthwhile mentioning these.

Inactivity

Disuse atrophy is an incontrovertible cause of bone loss. Other tissues besides bone decrease in mass, and the skeleton merely shows a response to the lack of stress that is occurring throughout the body. The mechanism is not understood but it is a local phenomenon and is self-limiting. Experimental studies mostly have been in denervated extremities. Studies in almost completely immobilized humans in bed rest have shown rapid bone loss (3). In paraplegics and quadriplegics, skeletal volume is significantly decreased. Other studies, on activity rather than immobilization, have shown a positive relationship between muscle mass and bone mass (4).

It is not easy to quantitate activity in older persons who are not hospitalized, but it is evident from even a superficial evaluation that the average older woman is considerably less active than a young person. The mechanism of the effect of exercise on bone is not precisely known but there is clearly an effect of stress on bone remodeling, tending to preserve bone and also probably to stimulate formation of new bone. Inactivity almost certainly contributes to senile osteoporosis.

Therefore, because disuse is a factor in osteoporosis, one facet of treatment is increased activity. For preventive therapy it would be reasonable to suggest an exercise regimen. However, it often is impossible to advise exercise, except in a mild form, to a patient who is suffering from this disease and has recently sustained a fracture, because additional fractures may result. Nevertheless, inactivity can be discouraged, and exercise can be advised as the skeleton responds to other forms of treament.

Protein Deficiency

By far the most important etiologic factor in osteoporosis appears to be nutrition. Because the skeleton is made up of calcium, phosphorus, and protein, it is these substances that must be considered in particular. Protein deficiency is a rare cause of osteoporosis; it occurs in the form of kwashiorkor in some scattered populations with unusual dietary habits and in some instances as a result of poverty and ignorance. The disease has been described in Africa and in the United States in Negro populations. In kwashiorkor, besides other manifestations of the disease such as irritability, there is a decrease in bone mass due to a failure of deposition of new tissue merely because amino acids are not available.

It is conceivable that a small number of elderly persons, particularly those living alone, may be protein-deficient to a minor extent; however, the average North American diet is more than adequate in its protein content and it is unlikely that lack of protein contributes significantly to the incidence of osteoporosis. However, if protein deficiency is noted in a patient's history, it is obvious that dietary counseling is necessary to correct this.

Vitamin C Deficiency

Scurvy is a documented cause of bone disease. It produces a failure of matrix formation and generally is accompanied by skin lesions. Vitamin C deficiency falls into the same category as protein deficiency in that it is rare, even in elderly patients. Any suspected vitamin C deficiency should be corrected by vitamin supplements.

Vitamin D Deficiency

This is an infrequent cause of rickets. As with calcium, the dietary requirements for vitamin D vary and the optimal level has not been established for all populations, although lack of vitamin D is becoming a well-recognized cause of both osteoporosis and osteomalacia in a specific population, the Asian immigrants to Great Britain. Their social habits lead them to remain indoors much of the time and, when they do go outside, they generally are heavily clothed. In addition, their diet contains little vitamin D but does contain significant quantities of phytates, which bind calcium. Their darker skin also decreases the natural synthesis of vitamin D that might result from what small exposure to sunlight they do have. Thus, social and dietary behaviors combine to make this population vitamin D deficient. Vitamin D deficiency can be corrected easily by the administration of relatively small amounts of vitamin D.

Abnormal Absorption of Vitamin D

Vitamin D may be present in an adequate amount in the diet and yet be inadequately absorbed in the intestine for a number of reasons. An obvious cause is complete or partial gastrectomy or any form of gastric surgery that decreases the site of vitamin D absorption. In addition, gastrectomy usually results in steatorrhea and a dumping syndrome, both of which would tend to cause vitamin D and also calcium to be lost. The importance of gastrectomy in the etiology of osteoporosis is substantiated in the literature; clinical evidence of osteomalacia, such as increased serum alkaline phosphatase, decreased serum calcium, and, in some instances, bone pain and pseudofractures, have been described in postgastrectomy patients. From the relationship between osteoporosis and osteomalacia, it is obvious that most postgastrectomy patients who develop osteomalacia also will have lost bone mass, and their symptoms will result from the combination of osteoporosis and osteomalacia. It would be reasonable to add both calcium and vitamin supplements to the diet of postgastrectomy patients.

Abnormalities of Vitamin D Metabolism

Any factor that interferes with the metabolism of vitamin D into its active forms will also decrease the gastrointestinal absorption of calcium. Such factors include extensive liver disease, anephric state, and the presence of substances such as phenobarbitone or diphosphonates. All can result in bone disease. Addition of the missing metabolite or its analog is the obvious form of treatment for such metabolic aberrations.

Calcium Deficiency

Relative insufficiency of vitamin D is a frequent cause of osteomalacia, if it is accepted that the lack of vitamin D does not mean only dietary lack of the hormone. The ultimate result is malabsorption of calcium, with bone disease secondary to calcium deficiency. If the dietary vitamin D level is normal and its metabolism is normal, it is virtually impossible to produce osteomalacia. In calcium deficiency, even rickets is rare. Calcium-containing fluid is exsorbed and endsorbed in the gastric and intestinal lumens so that, in instances of relatively low dietary calcium intake, absorption is adequate if sufficient vitamin D is present. Only if there is additional demand for or loss of calcium will a failure of mineralization occur and bone disease develop. The demand may be growth of new bone and the loss may be hypercalcemia, diarrhea, or other causes.

However, dietary calcium deficiency in the presence of normal levels of vitamin D may have an important role in the development of osteoporosis. Fecal calcium excretion generally is greater than urinary calcium excretion by a factor of 2, and the sum of both is greater than the dietary intake. The result is that most persons are in negative calcium balance for the major part of their adult lives. The skeleton supplies the calcium necessary to maintain the serum calcium concentration, bone is lost, and osteoporosis develops.

The daily requirement for calcium is not known; however, it may be suggested that dietary calcium intake is inadequate as long as there is a negative calcium balance. Calcium intake varies in different populations, and this variation may be responsible for the differences in incidence of osteoporosis. Because the majority of reports suggest that, in a population of persons of different ages, the bone mass decreases with age, the concept has developed that bone loss is an aging phenomenon. This may be true in general. However, carefully controlled longitudinal studies over an 11-year period have demonstrated that a significant number of persons did not lose bone mass (5). A high Singh index and a normal bone mass on biopsy in some older persons also strongly suggest that individuals may not lose bone to any great extent as they age. Presumably, these persons had an adequate calcium intake. Unfortunately, the longitudinal studies were not accompanied by dietary histories. However, independent investigations on ovolactovegetarians, omnivores, and exclusive carnivores (seal- and whale-eating Eskimos) do support this concept. Vegetarians who eat eggs and milk but avoid meat (a high-phosphorus food) have a higher bone density than omnivores; a population that eats only meat loses bone at a more rapid rate than omnivores (6, 7).

Studies in man and animals have raised the question of the role of calcium deficiency and phosphorus excess. In the United States the national diet is increasing in phosphorus content, but little attention is being paid to this trend. It is possible that the most important factor in the diet is the ratio of calcium to phosphorus. This has been suggested in animal studies in which normal bone density was maintained on both low and high phosphorus intakes, as long as the dietary calcium intake was higher than the phosphorus intake. Even on a relatively low calcium intake, if it is greater than the phosphorus intake, bone will not be lost.

Further work on this point should include relating dietary calcium and phosphorus levels in man with bone loss. A longitudinal study should show a more rapid loss in those in whom the calcium-to-phosphorus ratio is significantly less than 1. However, the major problem in such a study would be a much-needed reevaluation of the calcium and phosphorus contents of food. For example, an increasing number of persons eat processed cheese, which contains more phosphorus than calcium. A large number of other processed foods, such as ice cream and emulsion types of food, contain added phosphorus in the form of phosphate used to stabilize the emulsions. In addition to changes in the calcium and phosphorus contents of food, food-eating habits have changed considerably in the last 20 years. The consumption of snack foods, including crackers, potato chips, and soft drinks, has increased at least 200%; all these foods contain a high proportion of phosphorus. The per capita consumption of meat has also increased in the last 20 years by 31%, while that of dairy products has decreased 37%.

Another factor that results in increased phosphorus ingestion is the addition to food of chemicals such as orthophosphates (for acidifying food), diphosphonates (sometimes used to complex alkaline earth metals), and polyphosphates (which act to bind protein and complex calcium). These changes have occurred mainly over the last 10 years and have resulted in increased dietary intake of phosphorus and a decrease in calcium ingestion.

Phosphorus Excess

That phosphate excess will tend to exaggerate bone loss has been substantiated in animals and in population studies in man. In the animal studies, phosphate was added as a supplement in a neutral solution (8). In the epidemiologic investigations in man, the differences in phosphate content of the diet resulted from differences in the meat content of the diet, which ranged from 0 to nearly 100%.

Because it is the calcium-to-phosphorus ratio that appears to be important, it is not necessary to decrease the phosphorus intake if it is possible to increase the calcium intake. However, it is almost impossible to increase the calcium content of the diet enough to make the calcium-to-phosphorus ratio greater than 1 without calcium salt supplements. Milk and cheese contain only a small fraction more calcium than phosphorus, and other commonly eaten foods such as meat, bread, and potatoes are very high in phosphorus and contain little calcium. The majority of vegetables (excluding leafy vegetables) also contain more phosphorus than calcium. A very few, somewhat bizzare, types of food contain a large amount of calcium and little phosphorus; these include sesame seeds, molasses, and seaweed. These are not commonly eaten, and yet a high-calcium, low-phosphorus ingredient is precisely what is needed to offset the high-phosphorus, low-calcium content of most food.

In cases of phosphorus deprivation it is obvious that dietary phosphorus supplements are indicated until the serum phosphorus value is normal. However, the vast majority of people are not phosphorus depleted; in fact, they are eating too much phosphorus and are not able to correct this by reasonable means. It would be difficult to ingest only food with a calcium-to-phosphorus ratio higher than 1 (although this is the case among the blood- and milk-drinking Masai). Only by dietary calcium supplements can a correct calcium-to-phosphorus ratio be achieved.

Fluoride Excess

While preventive treatment is preferable, correction of osteoporosis is the primary problem. Because this disease may be expected to increase in incidence, it is reasonable to make efforts to "cure" it—that is, to induce an increase in bone mass. Calcium supplements and replacement of deficient hormones have not proved useful in increasing skeletal mass. Other forms of treatment, such as calcitonin or diphosphonates, have not shown promise yet and, at this time, fluoride appears to be the only substance known to stimulate osteoblasts and to cause the change in cellular behavior in bone that could achieve the increased mass essential for correction of the disorder.

Early studies with fluoride as the therapeutic agent in the treatment of osteoporosis were disappointing. The reason became evident from animal studies (9) in which high doses of fluoride resulted in a depression of serum calcium concentration, subsequent stimulation of parathyroid gland activity, and increased release of parathyroid hormone. Osteomalacia was also apparent on biopsy. The initial decrease in serum calcium could be explained by the increase in new bone, which resulted in a greater than usual demand for calcium.

Fluoride and Calcium

It has been demonstrated experimentally that the secondary hyperparathyroidism and hyperosteoidosis can be prevented by the oral administration of calcium supplements. Animal studies by Hauck and colleagues (10) in 1933 were perhaps the first to relate dietary history and fluoride levels to the bone structure. Later, in man, increased bone mass was seen in patients with multiple myeloma who had been treated with a combination of fluoride and calcium; cortisone-induced osteoporosis also responded favorably to treatment with fluoride and calcium (11). Presumably, the increased formation of new bone generates a need for additional calcium and this need can be satisfied by increased oral ingestion of calcium. In recent studies (12), vitamin D has been added to the combined fluoride and calcium regimen to increase the absorption of calcium, so that large calcium supplements are not necessary.

Two major questions had to be answered: the first was concerned with the optimal level of fluoride to produce a significant increase in bone formation and the second was related to toxicity. To answer the first question, patients were given different levels of fluoride, from 30 mg to 90 mg of sodium fluoride per day (15 to 45 mg of fluoride). The level of supplemental calcium was also varied to find the amount necessary for calcification of new bone and for suppression of hyperparathyroidism. The preliminary studies suggested that 50 mg of sodium fluoride per day (25 mg of fluoride) and 1 g of calcium per day as an oral supplement (the carbonate form appears satisfactory) is an effective combination; 50,000 units of vitamin D were also given twice a week. Further investigation is needed at this time to decide if this is the optimal dose or if vitamin D is required at all. Of the three components of the treatment regimen, the vitamin D is potentially the most toxic because it can produce hypercalcemia and hypercalciuria and can endanger renal function.

The roentgenographic appearance of fluoride-treated persons may be described as "fluorosis" in that there is coarsening of trabeculae and increased density of bone as a result of increased amounts of bone.

However, the term "fluorosis" is most frequently used to describe the total picture seen in areas where there are increased amounts of fluoride in the drinking water and where persons have been exposed to the high fluoride content all their lives. In the Punjab region of India, the amount of fluoride in the drinking water varies from 1.4 to 9.7 mg/liter; because it is hard to estimate the amount of water drunk in this area it is not possible to estimate the total dose received per person. However, it is possible to say that the dose may range from 2.0 mg/day, which would not be expected to produce an effect on bone (and, in fact, does not), to 40 mg/day or more, which would be above the therapeutic dose recommended by our studies in osteoporotic humans.

The dose based on ingestion of drinking water is obviously an underestimate because it does not include the fluoride in the food and the recirculation of fluoride from the bone. It is most likely, therefore, that the clinical manifestations of fluorosis, such as mottled teeth, periosteal exostoses, and consequent neurologic complaints, occur at higher levels of fluoride ingestion than those suggested as therapeutic levels and that the symptoms result largely from the fact that the affected persons have ingested fluoride all their lives.

In the Punjab studies by Jolly (13), the calcium content of the water appeared to modify the effects of fluoride on the skeleton, the incidence of fluorosis increasing nearly fivefold in some areas having soft water. The hardness of drinking water in the United States is higher than that of the soft-water Punjab villages and, with the dietary calcium supplements suggested in our regimen, the incidence of neurologic complications resulting from fluoride ingestion should be almost negligible. The mechanism of the effect of calcium on fluoride absorption is not fully known; a tenfold increase in calcium intake will cause a twofold decrease in fluoride absorption because of the formation of insoluble calcium fluoride. This accounts for some of the effect on absorption but does not explain it all.

Experience is still needed on the unwanted side-effects of long-term fluoride and calcium treatment of osteoporotic patients. After 5 years of investigation, periosteal exostosis has occurred in one patient (a bony spur developed at the site of the bone biopsy, probably as the result of the trauma of the biopsy and the fluoride-induced overstimulated healing at the biopsy site). The two most frequent adverse effects were gastric discomfort and joint pain. The gastric pain generally can be prevented by giving the fluoride with meals. Swelling and pain in the joints, particularly the knees, is reversible on withdrawal of the fluoride and may not recur when treatment is continued. Fluoride has been shown to stimulate the fibroblast system and hasten connective tissue formation in healing (14), a not-unexpected finding in view of its influence on osteoblasts, which are derived from the fibroblast system. At the lower levels achieved in the osteoporosis treatment regimen, occasional stimulation of the synovial membrane appears to occur and cause discomfort. In only one person (3%) has fluoride had to be withdrawn completely because of joint pain and swelling.

CONCLUSIONS

From what is now known of the factors that contribute to the etiology of osteoporosis, it is becoming apparent that symptomatic disease will occur more frequently in the future, particularly if general medical care improves and more people live longer. Prevention of symptomatic osteoporosis is theoretically possible by correcting the deficiencies that contribute to the bone loss. Calcium supplements will restore the calcium-to-phosphorus ratio to normal—greater than 1. Exercise will increase bone mass, and estrogen replacement should be considered in estrogen-deprived patients. However, prevention is not always possible because it is difficult to treat persons for a disease they do not have but may develop. The problem is that it would be reasonable to treat the process of bone loss by using preventive therapy, but the symptoms occur only as an end-stage of this process, and that is too late for preventive treatment. A combined regimen of fluoride and calcium is the form of treatment necessary for patients with the disease who have not been treated prophylactically.

A number of questions are almost always evoked by a discussion of fluoride as a therapeutic agent. The fluoridation of drinking water or the ingestion of high-fluoride foods, such as tea, fish, or salt, is an unreliable source of fluoride if therapy is being considered. An unreasonable volume of fluoridated water would have to be drunk, and tea, fish, or salt would have to be eaten daily in large quantities in order to achieve a therapeutic level. Only in areas where the water content is naturally high, such as parts of Texas and North and South Dakota, would it be possible to obtain an oral intake that approximated the therapeutic dose. It might be expected that people from these areas should never become osteoporotic. However, it cannot be stressed too emphatically that the success of the fluoride treatment depends on the accompanying calcium. In fact, fluoride alone would eventually cause a net loss of skeletal mass unless calcium supplements were used.

It also is apparent that correct dietary calcium levels would be a first and most important step toward preventing osteoporosis and that the fluoride and calcium regimen may prove to be an effective form of treatment once symptomatic bone disease is present. Fluoride is still considered an investigational new drug. Further studies in larger groups and evaluation of the side-effects and complications of this therapy are currently being carried out (15).

REFERENCES

1. Barnett, E. and Nordin, B. E. C. *Clin Radiol.* **11:**166 (1960).
2. Singh, M., Riggs, B. L., Beaubout, J. W., and Jowsey, J. *Ann. Intern. Med.* **77:**63 (1972).
3. Donaldson, C. L., Hulley, S. B., Vogel, J. M., Hattner, R. S., Bayers, J. H., and McMillan, D. E. *Metab. Clin. Exp.* **19:**1071 (1970).
4. Doyle, F., Brown, J., and Lachance, C. *Lancet* **1:**391 (1970).
5. Adams, P., Davies, G. T., and Sweetnam, P. *Quart. J. Med.* **39:**601 (1970).
6. Ellis, F. R., Holesh, S., and Ellis, J. W. *Am. J. Clin. Nutr.* **25:**555 (1972).
7. Mazess, R. B. *Arctic Anthropol.* **7:**114 (1970).
8. Laflamme, G. H., and Jowsey, J. *J. Clin. Invest.* **51:**2834 (1972).
9. Faccini, J. M., and Care, A. D. *Nature* (London) **207:**1399 (1965).
10. Hauck, H. M., Steenbock, H., and Parsons, H. T. *Am. J. Physiol.* **103:**489 (1933).
11. Cohen, P., Nichols, G. L., Jr., and Banks, H. H. *Clin. Orthop.* **64:**221 (1969).
12. Jowsey, J., Riggs, B. L., Kelly, P. J., and Hoffman, D. L. *Am. J. Med.* **53:**43 (1972).
13. Jolly, S. S. (1970) Hydric fluorosis in Punjab (India). In *Fluoride in Medicine* T. L. Vischer, Ed., Hans Huber, Bern, 1970, pp. 106-121.
14. Joseph, J. and Tydd, M. *Nature* (London) **246:**165 (1973).
15. Jowsey, J., Riggs, B. L., and Kelly, P. J. *Postgrad. Med.* **52:**62 (1972).

8

Periodontal Disease

LEO LUTWAK

Veterans Administration Hospital, Sepulveda, California

What is the interest of periodontal disease, a dental disorder, to the physician and nutritionist? Periodontal disease is responsible for the loss of teeth in approximately 35 million people in this country (1), most of whom are in the category considered aged. Edentulous patients suffer from malnutrition because without teeth it is impossible to eat a normal diet, and even with optimal replacement the palatability of food decreases, also contributing to malnutrition. As a result, the aged individual who is edentulous and has poorly fitting dentures changes his pattern of eating, consuming more of soft, high-carbohydrate foods.

A second reason for considering periodontal disease arises from the studies in the past 20 years of osteoporosis and related disorders of bone demineralization. Data from many laboratories, including our own, suggest that bone demineralization is the result of chronic dietary deficiency of calcium and chronic dietary excess of phosphorus, conditions extremely prevalent in our society (2).

Among other factors that have been suggested as contributing to osteoporosis are relative estrogen deficiency, and immobilization. The role of estrogen secretion is probably minimal. Women, who secrete estrogen throughout their entire adult lives, also have less bone than men throughout their adult lives. Hence, it is apparent that under normal physiologic conditions estrogen does not lead to increased new bone formation and therefore is not responsible primarily for skeletal mineralization. Furthermore, in therapeutic trials, when estrogens are administered in large amounts for long periods of time to postmenopausal women, there is little, if any, effect on the total retention of calcium by the skeleton (3–6).

Total immobilization leads to rapid skeletal loss of calcium. This was

145

demonstrated in studies of immobilized volunteers (7) and, more dramatically, in astronauts under zero gravity (8). However, the effect is seen only with total immobilization and is readily reversed by minimal gravitational stress.

Recent studies have led to the conclusion that the primary factor in the development of osteoporosis in patients free of endocrine and gastrointestinal disorders is chronic dietary deficiency of calcium associated with excess dietary phosphorus. Furthermore, this phenomenon may also be responsible for a significant proportion of periodontal disease.

The recommended daily allowances for calcium and phosphorus of the Food and Nutrition Board of the National Research Council is 800 milligrams per day of each for the adult (9) (Table 1). It should be emphasized that the recommended daily allowances represent the best educated guesses based on published information for the amount of the nutrient that will protect the majority of the population from disease. Particularly when considering requirements for elements such as calcium and phosphorus, one must remember that these recommended allowances are based on limited numbers of studies of varying validity. On the other hand, recommended allowances for various animal species other than man are generally based on considerably

Table 1   Recommended Daily Allowances[a]

	Age	Calcium	Phosphorus	Ca/P
	(yr)	(mg)	(mg)	
Infants	0 - 0.5	360	240	1.5
	0.5 - 1.0	540	400	1.35
Children	1 - 10	800	800	1.0
Males	11 - 18	1200	1200	1.0
	19+	800	800	1.0
Females	11 - 18	1200	1200	1.0
	19+	800	800	1.0
Pregnant		1200	1200	1.0
Lactating		1200	1200	1.0

[a]Data from (9).

Table 2   Recommended Daily Allowances for Different Species

Animal	Weight (kg)	Calcium (mg/kg)	Phosphorus (mg/kg)	Ca/P	Reference
Cattle	636	17	17	1.0	10a
Horse	636	20	20	1.0	10b
Swine	227	90	60	1.5	10c
Sheep	73	52	42	1.24	10d
Man	70	11	11	1.0	9
Dog	50	62	52	1.2	10e
	10	95	79	1.2	
	1	175	146	1.2	

larger numbers of studies. It is of interest (see Table 2) to see the considerable variation in order of magnitude between man and other more carefully studied animals.

Food disappearance data from statistics published by the United States Department of Agriculture (Table 3) (11) indicate that in 1957 an average of 383 grams of calcium per year and 1073 grams of phosphorus per year were "consumed" in the United States for each person. True consumption was significantly less because these data do not allow for plate waste and nonhuman consumption. The calcium/phosphorus ratio in this available diet was about 1:3. Most of the calcium intake came from milk and milk products, with small amounts obtained from baked goods made with fortified flour and from fruits and vegetables. The phosphorus in the American diet came partly from milk but also, in large amounts, from meat, poultry, fish, and flour. Since these data were obtained, there have been significant changes in the American dietary pattern (12). Milk consumption has been decreasing by an average of 10% per year. Furthermore, because of the improved standard of living of the average person, there has been an increase in meat consumption, leading to an increase in phosphorus intake. In addition, elimination of milk from the diet has been accompanied by increased consumption of other beverages, particularly soft drinks. As demonstrated in Table 4, soft drink consumption in the United States has been increasing in a geometric fashion (13). In 1850, the first year for which data are available, the average consumption was 1 eight ounce container per person per year. By 1920

Table 3   Annual Per Capita Food Disappearance in the United States[a]

Food Category	Calcium (g)	Phosphorus (g)
Bakery products	37.0	75
Whole grain products	10.0	50
Flour	8.6	100
Macaroni	0.7	5
Rice	1.1	6
Potatoes	5.8	30
Root Vegetables	6.1	6
Fresh vegetables	15.0	50
Canned vegetables	4.2	10
Dried beans	2.9	10
Fresh fruit	13.6	20
Canned fruit	1.3	2
Fruit juices	1.7	2
Meat	10.9	200
Poultry	9.2	140
Fish	10.8	130
Eggs	9.1	36
Shellfish	0.8	1
Milk products	234.3	200
Total	383	1073
Ratio	1 to	2.8

[a] Data from (11).

this had increased to 38; after World War II, in 1946, the figure was 132. By 1973, the average consumption of soft drinks was 430 eight-ounce containers per year per person. About 60% of this was in the form of cola beverages (14). Recent unpublished analyses from our laboratory (15) have shown that the calcium content of soft drinks is extremely low, about 2 to 5 mg/100 ml, generally related to the calcium content of the local water supply. The phosphorus content of cola beverages is between 12 and 20 mg %, while that of the other flavors is generally lower. Thus, at the present time, in our soft drink consuming generation, calcium intake has been decreasing, while phosphorus intake has been increasing.

The effect of dietary calcium inadequacy can be demonstrated by a simple calculation. Let us consider a typical patient. Since diseases of demineralization are more common in women, this patient is a 50-year-old woman who weighs 55 kg. At age 20 she weighed about the same, with a total body calcium content of about 1800 g. Diet surveys of middle class American adult women have indicated a usual calcium intake of about 400 mg/day. Studies of calcium absorption at this intake level have demonstrated a range of 5 to 50% efficiency, with a mode at about 35% (16). For this calculation let us assume 45% efficiency. resulting in an absorption of 180 mg/day. Urinary calcium excretion ranges from 100 to 200 mg for the normal adult. Endogenous fecal excretion ranges from 140 to 175 mg/day. Assuming 100 mg for urinary loss and 150 mg for fecal loss, and adding an additional 20 mg/day for losses of desquamated skin and sweat, we arrive at 270 mg/day of total losses. Thus, this person has been in negative balance for an average of 90 mg/day for the 30 years under consideration, more than sufficient to produce significant skeletal demineralization.

Table 4 Estimated Annual Per Capita Consumption of Soft Drinks[a]

Year	Per Capita (8-oz containers)
1849	1.6
1869	6.4
1889	9.9
1909	16.2
1919	38.4
1929	53.1
1939	88.6
1945	132.9
1950	158.0
1952	174.0
1955	184.2
1958	186.4
1960	192.0
1963	227.4
1965	259.1
1967	298.1
1969	344.4
1971	388.1
1972	406.4
1973	429.6

[a] Data from (13).

This loss has developed gradually, over the course of many years, and is sufficient to account for the degrees of osteoporosis seen in women between ages 50 and 60 without requiring consideration of the acute effects of menopause.

When patients with established osteoporosis are placed on diets containing the same calcium and phosphorus contents as their usual intakes and complete metabolic balance studies of 30 to 50 days are carried out, these patients are found to be in negative calcium balance with continuing loss of this element (17). If calcium intake is then increased stepwise, with 1- to 2-month adaptation to new intake and repeated long-term balance studies at the new levels, more retention of calcium is seen as the intakes increase. Although it has been repeatedly demonstrated that the efficiency of absorption of calcium decreases with increasing intake, the absolute amount of calcium absorbed increases until intakes of the order of 1500 to 2000 mg/day are reached. When balance studies are repeated after several years of high intake, it has been found that the degree of positive calcium balance diminishes with time (18). The interpretation of this observation has been that in patients with established osteoporosis the potential for remineralization is diminished because of the occurrence of fractures and the loss of tissue where remineralization can occur. The implication of this is that once vertebral collapse has occurred, osteoporosis may be halted but cannot be reversed. Hence for prevention of irreversible collapse and fracture, it becomes essential to find early diagnostic signs of osteoporosis and institute therapy before the point of irreversibility has been reached.

Studies have been conducted with animal models in collaboration with Professor Lennart Krook of the New York State Veterinary College at Cornell University. Skeletal demineralization, radiographically and histologically similar to human osteoporosis, has been developed in monkeys (19), cats (20), horses (21), and dogs (22). In all species, the findings of osteoporosis have appeared after the administration of diets low in calcium and high in phosphorus.

In a prospective study with adult beagles (22), generalized osteoporosis was developed by feeding a diet with a calcium/phosphorus ratio of 1:10. Both the experimental diet and the control diet (with a calcium/phosphorus ratio of 1.2:1) were identical in consistency. Increased bone resorption was found on histologic examination of all bones. Clinically, the first lesions detected were areas of demineralization in the alveolar bone of the mandible. Resorption of trabecular bone in this tissue led to loosening of the teeth, followed by traumatization of the gingivae, followed in turn by exudation, hemorrhage,

and superinfection of the gums, a picture identical to human periodontal disease. Examination of the parathyroid glands of these animals
demonstrated relative hypersecretion in the animals on high-
phosphorus, calcium-deficient diets—nutritional secondary hyperparathyroidism.

A second study (23) demonstrated that the lesions of demineralization, both in the long bones and in the jaws, were reversible by refeed-
ing the animals diets with high-calcium, normal phosphorus content,
with a calcium/phosphorus ratio of 1.2:1 for approximately 42 weeks.
Demineralization of the jaw occurred at about the same rate as in the
vertebrae, both much more rapid than in the long bones. Similarly,
remineralization was more rapid and more complete in the jaw and
vertebrae than in the long bones. These observations suggested that
osteoporosis of the jaw, with associated periodontal disease, might be
an early form of generalized nutritional osteoporosis.

Retrospective observations in patients with periodontal disease confirmed the coincident appearance of vertebral osteoporosis and
periodontal disease (24). Most patients with severe axial osteoporosis
were edentulous. Patients with mild osteoporosis had significant degrees of periodontal disease and alveolar bone resorption.

Histologically, human periodontal disease resembled the experimental observations in the dogs. Examination of parathyroid glands of
patients who died of other causes with coincidental periodontal disease
and osteoporosis similarly showed foci of hyperplastic secretory cells.

The hypothesis that human periodontal disease might, in part, be a
form of nutritional osteoporosis was tested in a pilot study with 90
unselected patients (25, 26). Each patient received either placebo or
calcium supplement sufficient to provide an additional 1.0 gram of
calcium per day for 6 months or 12 months. Patients were evaluated
monthly by blood and urine analyses for calcium and phosphorus and
by measurements of bone density using photondensitometry (27) of the
radius, ulna, and os mentis.

No changes were seen in any patients in blood or urinary content of
any of the elements measured. No significant changes were seen in
bone density of any of the bones measured in the groups evaluated for
6 months. In the patients receiving treatment for 12 months, no significant differences were seen in the density of either the radius of the
ulna between the placebo and calcium-supplemented groups. However,
marked changes were seen in the os mentis. There was no significant
change noted in the group receiving placebo. The group receiving 1.0
gram of calcium per day as a dietary supplement showed an average of
12% increase in bone density over the 12-month evaluation period.

This was significant at p < 0.001.

This study is currently being repeated with a larger number of patients, who are receiving either calcium, calcium plus fluoride, or placebo, on a double-blind basis for 18 months. In addition to bone density evaluations, periodontal evaluations are being performed at 6-month intervals. From these studies, three questions may be answered. *(1)* Is periodontal disease an early form of osteoporosis? *(2)* Can periodontal disease be reversed (and therefore osteoporosis as well) by dietary calcium supplementation? *(3)* Does fluoride, when added to calcium, improve the rate or the amount of remineralization that can occur?

REFERENCES

1.   Anonymous. Need for dental care among adults, United States, 1960-1962. National Center for Health Statistics, Series 11, No. 36. U.S.D.H.E.W., Public Health Service, Washington, D.C., 1970.

2.   Lutwak, L. *Geriatrics* **29**:171 (1974).

3.   Lutwak, L. and Whedon, G. D. *Fed. Proc.* **22**:553 (1963).

4.   Lutwak, L. Effects of estrogens and androgens in metabolic bone disease. Abstr. Second Internat. Congr. Hormonal Steroids 329 (1966).

5.   Riggs, B. L., Jowsey, J., Goldsmith, R. S., Kelly, P. J., Hoffman, D. L., and Arnaud, C. D. *J. Clin. Invest.* **51**:1659 (1972).

6.   Ruikka, I., Gronroos, M., Sourander, L. B., and Virtama, P. *Geriatrics* **23**:165 (1963).

7.   Deitrick, J. E., Whedon, G. D., and Shorr, E. *Am. J. Med.* **4**:3 (1948).

8.   Lutwak, L., Whedon, G. D., Lachance, P. A., Reid, J. M., and Lipscomb, H. S. *J. Clin. Endocrinol. Metab.* **29**:1140 (1969).

9.   Committee on Dietary Allowances. Recommended dietary allowances, Eighth Edition. National Academy of Sciences. Washington, D.C., 1974.

10.   a. Nutrient requirements for cattle. National Research Council No. 3 (1962).
       b. Nutrient requirements for horses. National Research Council No. 6 (1962).
       c. Nutrient requirements for swine. National Research Council No. 2 (1962).
       d. Nutrient requirements for sheep. National Research Council No. 5 (1962).
       e. Nutrient requirements for dogs. National Research Council No. 8 (1962).

11.   Dietary levels of households in the United States. U.S. Household Food Consumption Survey, 1955. U.S.D.A. Report No. 6. Washington, D.C., 1972.

12.   Food and nutrient intake of individuals in the United States, Spring 1965. U.S.D.A. Report No. 11. Washington, D.C., 1972.

13.   1973 Sales Survey of the soft drink industry. National Soft Drink Assoc., Washington, D.C., 1973.

14.   Bacon, R. Soft drinks. In *U.S. Industrial Outlook, 1974, with projections to 1980.* U.S.D. of Commerce, Washington, D.C., 1974.

15.   Lutwak, L. and Cochran, V. Mineral content of soft drinks. To be published.

16.   Lutwak, L. *Am. J. Clin. Nutr.* **22**:771 (1969).

17.   Lutwak, L. and Whedon, G. D. Osteoporosis. Disease-a-Month, April, 1963.

18.   Lutwak, L. *J. Am. Diet. Assoc.* **44:**173 (1964).

19.   Krook, L. and Barrett, R. B. *Cornell Vet.* **52:**459 (1962).

20.   Krook, L., Barrett, R. B., Usui, K., and Wolke, R. E. *Cornell Vet.* **53:**224 (1963).

21.   Krook, L. and Lowe, J. E. *Pathol. Vet.* **1:** (Suppl.) 71 (1961).

22.   Henrikson, P. A. *Acta Odont. Scand.* **26** (Suppl): 50 (1968).

23.   Krook, L., Lutwak, L., Henrikson, P. A., Kallfelz, F., Hirsch, C., Romanus, B., Belanger, L. F., Marier, J. R., and Sheffy, B. E. *J. Nutr.* **101:**233 (1971).

24.   Krook, L., Lutwak, L., Whalen, J. P., Henrikson, P. A., Lesser, G. V., and Uris, R. *Cornell Vet.* **62:**32 (1972).

25.   Lutwak, L., Krook, L., Whalen, J., and Coulston, A. *Israel J. Med. Sci.* **7:**504 (1971).

26.   Lutwak, L. and Coulston, A. Dietary calcium and the jaw bone. In International Conference on Bone Mineral Measurement, 1973. R. Mazess, Ed. DHEW Publication No. 75-683, Washington, D.C., 1975, p. 285.

27.   Cameron, J. R. and Sorenson, J. *Science* **142:**230 (1963).

9

The Role of Fiber in the Diet

THOMAS P. ALMY, M.D.

Dartmouth Medical School, Hanover, New Hampshire

Urbanization and the habitation of temperate and subarctic zones, two striking characteristics of Western culture, have been viewed by many as linked to a drastic change in diet in that culture in the last 100 to 150 years. The need to store food for long periods of time between harvests, and the smaller bulk and longer shelf-life of refined sugars and cereal grains, have led to increasing consumption of these products and a declining intake of crude vegetable fiber. The more affluent have compensated for this with their salad bowls, but have offset this advantage in turn by greater consumption of meat and dairy products.

Recently, the suspicion has grown that certain gastrointestinal conditions of high or clearly increasing prevalence in our society are attributable in part to deficiency of dietary fiber (Table 1). The evidence for an etiologic role for fiber deficiency in these diseases includes epidemiologic, clinical, physiologic, and biochemical observations, and in some instances experimental reproduction in laboratory animals. In other instances, the attribution is merely speculative or based on anecdote. Many observations, though confirmed, are not unchallenged. Therefore a brief review at this time had better serve as a background for further inquiry rather than as a blueprint for health policy.

CONDITIONS ATTRIBUTABLE TO LACK OF FIBER

Constipation

In placing chronic constipation at the top of the list, I am referring to two established effects of dietary fiber—first that the amount of it is positively correlated with the size of the stools, and second that this

155

Table 1   Digestive Diseases and Disorders Attributed in Part to Deficiency of Dietary Vegetable Fiber 1974

Chronic constipation
Diverticular disease of the colon
Carcinoma of the colon
Cholelithiasis
Hiatus hernia
Hemorrhoids
Appendicitis

amount is inversely related to the time required for evacuation of residues (1-3). By the simple expedient of feeding plastic pellets with the regular diet to a group of English boys in a public school and to the inhabitants of an African village, Burkitt (Table 2) was able to recognize a marked difference in passage time inversely related to stool bulk (4,5). In several studies this relationship of stool mass to transit time was consistent (Fig. 1). This correlation, of course, is attributed to cumulative absorption of fecal water with longer retention in the colon; and older impressions of the significance of this delayed passage time in constipated individuals have been recently confirmed by modern methods of measurement of absorption from the lumen (3).

The relief of constipation by restoration of bulk to the diet has been documented for more than thirty years by a mass of reports of clinical improvement after use of bran or cellulose/hemi-cellulose preparations, much of the evidence being without controls but some reasonably

Table 2   Two Populations: An English Boarding School Compared with an African Village[a]

	English School	African Village
Daily average weight of stool (g)	113	452
Average passage time of stool (hr)	80	30

[a]Data from (4).

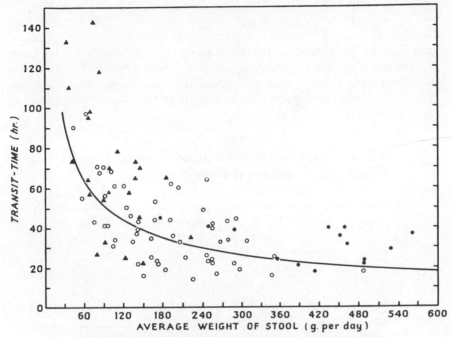

Relation between fibre intake, transit-time, and stool weight.
O = Vegetarians, vegans, and African boarding-school (mixed diet).
● = African villagers (high-residue diet).
▲ = English boarding-school and British Navy (low-residue diet).
The curve (which is based on more data than the points shown here) is:
    log (time) = 2·81633–0·56057 log (weight).

Figure 1.   Relation between stool weight and transit time in several groups of subjects on diets of widely varying content of vegetable fiber. From (5).

satisfactory. Stool weights have been again carefully studied and shown to increase as the result of such treatment. Thus this very common ailment, undoubtedly influenced by many factors, and undoubtedly one of the curses of the aged in our society, can be related in part to our refined diet. Correction of fiber deficiency is one of the more manageable aspects of the problem.

Diverticular Disease

Diverticular disease of the colon is a major cause of disability in the elderly. Though we have no adequate survey of its prevalence in the United States, it is probable that disability from this cause affects between 5 and 10% of our population over 60 years of age; its prevalence in asymptomatic form is four or five times higher.

This is clearly an acquired, age-related condition. The data collected by Manousos and Truelove at Oxford (Table 3) indicate the rapid increase in prevalence with increasing age. They fed barium to unselected outpatients attending *all* clinics at the Radcliffe Infirmary, and used only a single roentgenogram for each person (6). It appears to be increasing in frequency more rapidly even than the proportion of aged persons in our population.

Table 3   Prevalence of Diverticulosis in the General Population, Radiological Survey[a]

Age	No. of Subjects	No. with Diverticula	Prevalence (%)
Under 40	39	0	0.0
40–59	27	5	18.5
60–79	24	7	29.2
Over 80	19	8	42.1

[a]Data modified from (6).

Most striking differences in the frequency of this condition have been reported (7) between developed Westernized countries and the developing countries of the tropics (Table 4). Yet the correlation is not with the level of modernization, for the prevalence figures in Japan and Korea are low. Though these differences might be attributed to racial or genetic factors, the prevalence appears to be much higher, for example, among blacks in Harlem or even in Kinshasa than among their distant cousins in rural Africa. Some Japanese physicians have told me that every time they come for an extended stay in the United States, their stools get smaller. All of these observations seem best fitted to a hypothesis involving one or more major environmental factors, and the most widely held view is that the principal factor is fiber deficiency in the diet of the United States, Northern Europe, and other highly developed countries with a long food pipeline from producer to consumer. The hypothesis is further supported by the experimental production of colonic diverticula in aging laboratory animals—including the rat (8,9) and the rabbit (10)—consuming diets unnaturally low in fiber.

Table 4   Incidence of Diverticulitis in Various Populations[a]

Country	Population Served		Mean Age	Diverticulitis Cases/10^6/Year
Scotland	European	400,000	68	12.88
Nigeria	African	400,000	53	0.17
Singapore	European	15,000	59	5.41
	Chinese	1,014,000	58	0.14
	Malay	190,500	53	0.10
	Indian	111,000	49	0.18
Fiji	European	7,500	60	7.62
	Indian	165,000	51	0.34

[a]Data modified from (7).

If this association is valid, how can it be explained? These are pulsion diverticula, really herniations of mucosa and submucosa through the circular muscle layer of the colon to lie beneath the serosa, 90% of them being in the sigmoid colon. The essential condition, aside from the presence of small defects in that muscle layer, is *increased intraluminal pressure*; or better, an increased *gradient* of pressure between lumen and peritoneal cavity, which can only be produced by contraction of the intrinsic musculature of the colon. Though not all agree with Arfwidsson (Table 5) that the resting pressure is elevated, the increased response to stimulation by food, neostigmine, and (in the hands of others) morphine is widely confirmed (11).

I have asserted that stool mass is in part a function of dietary fiber intake, and I submit that in a *filled* segment of colon stool mass is a

Table 5   Sigmoid Motility Studies, "Total Pressure"[a]

	Normal	Diverticular Disease
Basal	10.77 ± 3.3	56.61 ± 10.6
After eating	31.57 ± 5.0	174.81 ± 25.3
Neostigmine	53.08 ± 10.6	177.87 ± 17.4

[a]Data from (11).

determinant of the *diameter* of the bowel. Diameter (or colon radius) can be related to the intraluminal pressure. If we begin with the law of Young and Laplace, we find that

$$T = k\,PR$$

This applies of course to the distension of a cylinder from within by an applied pressure P, with T (tension) as the dependent variable. But in the normally contractile gut tension is generated by muscular contraction, and pressure becomes the dependent variable. If we solve for pressure, we find

$$P = k \cdot \frac{T}{R},$$

or for any given level of muscle contraction the pressure generated is inversely related to the radius (or diameter) of the bowel.

This would suggest that increasing the size of the fecal mass by feeding bran or cellulose would yield lower sigmoidal pressures, especially during the increased activity induced by food or neostigmine. Findlay and his associates have found some evidence for this after five weeks of dietary supplementation with bran, 20 g daily (3). Hodgson (Table 6) found similar and more striking effects after six months of treating six patients with diverticular disease with methylcellulose tablets (12).

The clinical results of increasing the fiber intake of patients with diverticular disease have been generally gratifying, though only a single

Table 6   Sigmoid Motility before and after Methylcellulose Treatment[a]

| | Colonic Motility Index | | |
	Before	After	p
Resting	7577	1236	< 0.025
During feeding	13592	2645	< 0.01
Postprandial	8237	1761	< 0.05

[a]Data from (12).

properly controlled clinical trial has been reported (13) in preliminary fashion. Such evidence is badly needed, for the authors of many textbooks still recommend a low-residue diet for this disease, based, it would seem, on the finding of vegetable skins and seeds in the diverticula at operation or autopsy, and the supposition that these may induce diverticulitis through physical injury to the mucosa. Painter, on the other hand, has reported excellent clinical results (14) from feeding bran to such patients, and the unrecorded experience of many clinicians with psyllium seed and other cellulose preparations strongly supports the fiber deficiency hypothesis and indicates that this aspect of the disease may be readily manageable.

Carcinoma of the Colon

Cancer of the colon (including the rectum) is the next, and certainly the most important, disease on my list of digestive conditions related to diet. It is *the most common internal cancer* of United States citizens. Despite great advances in clinical diagnosis and surgical management over the past 40 years, it still accounts for nearly 50,000 *deaths* per year, in which respect it is exceeded only by carcinoma of the lung. It is clearly a disease of advancing age; its frequency rises steeply beyond age 40. Except for associations with some rare entities such as familial polyposis of the colon, genetic influences on its causation appear to be minor, and environmental influence correspondingly great.

As with diverticular disease, international comparisons of prevalence figures reveal striking differences and suggest a strong correlation with economic development, Western style (Fig. 2). The United States and Canada lead the world in prevalence, and the resident of Hartford, Connecticut, for example, has about 15 times the risk of developing this disease of a resident of the same age in Kampala, Uganda (15). Again, these differences cannot be reasonably attributed to racial or genetic factors. As Haenszel and his associates first showed us, among groups that immigrate to our country from regions of much lower prevalence, the risk of colonic cancer rises within ten years or so to approximately that of the native born population of the United States (16). This is particularly striking among the Japanese migrants to Hawaii and California (17), for their now highly industrialized homeland has been one of the conspicuous exceptions to the rule relating the frequency of colon cancer to economic development.

To what characteristic of Western civilization can this disease be attributed? The epidemiologists have provided us with a fairly refined and testable hypothesis. Drasar and Irving, for example, reported last year from the London School of Hygiene (18) on the correlation of

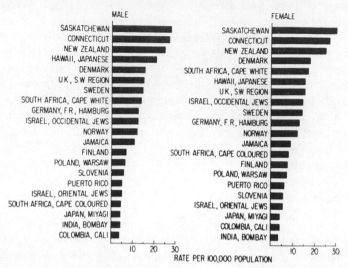

Figure 2. Prevalence of carcinoma of the colon in various national and ethnic groups. From (15).

colon cancer rates in 37 countries, with a number of variables related in one way or another to economic development (Table 7). Although correlations were found with such seemingly remote factors as per capita income, motorcars, radios, and TV sets, the stronger correlations were with dietary factors, and their predominance was reaffirmed by multiple regression analysis in which the contribution of nondietary factors could be mathematically eliminated. Note that the most significant coefficients are for so-called combined fat (which excludes cooking oils, butter, and the like) and animal protein, and that here very little influence appears for sugar and sweets versus fiber-rich carbohydrate sources.

The effect of the American diet on the probability of developing colonic cancer can be manifested in a number of ways. First of all, the fecal residue left by a diet that derives most of its calories from fat and protein, and that furnishes carbohydrate chiefly in the form of simple sugars and refined cereals, is going to be small, and its transit time delayed. Thus if an intraluminal carcinogen is truly operative, this kind of diet will present it over a longer period of time and in higher concentration to the epithelial surface of the colon.

Although these factors of time and concentration are probably significant, the complex chemical interrelationships of fiber residues, constituents of bile, end products of bacterial metabolism, and ingested carcinogens appear to be even more so. Some chemically defined substances that produce colonic cancers predictably in experimental animals have been shown by Weisburger (19) and others to be a useful model of these probable interactions in the induction of cancer in man. For example, a palm nut glycoside, cycasin, after initial absorption from the intestine, is transformed by a series of enzymatic processes of the liver cell, and subsequently of the colonic flora, into a much more potent carcinogen. Since colonic cancer can be produced experimentally by agents as diverse as the cycasins, the nitrosamines, and the polycyclic hydrocarbons, and since the complexities of metabolic events in the colonic lumen defy description, no one in his right mind would today suggest that a single carcinogen is responsible for the high endemicity of this tumor in our population.

For a variety of reasons, nevertheless, the role of *bile acids* (or bile salts) is today of intense interest. The sterol nucleus of bile acids can be dehydrogenated by four different enzymatic reactions, all of which can be produced by bacteria from the human colon, and three of which can be accomplished by the same group of Clostridia (20,21). The end-product is a phenanthrene compound of established carcinogenicity. Even one of these reactions yields deoxycholic acid, the most abundant secondary bile acid and itself a weak carcinogen; and as Hill and his

Table 7 Environmental Factors and Cancer of the Colon, Correlation Coefficients[a]

Dietary Factors		Nondietary Factors	
Combined fat	+ 0.87		
Animal protein	0.86		
Animal fat	0.80		
Total fat	0.77		
		Vehicles	+ 0.75
Eggs	0.73		
Total protein	0.70		
		Annual income	0.69
		Radios	0.59
Sugar and sweets	0.30		
		TV sets	0.25
Vegetable fiber	0.03		

[a]Approximate values, from Fig. 3 of (18).

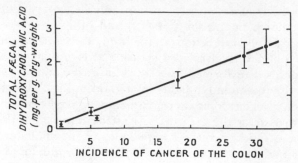

Figure 3. Relation between incidence of carcinoma of the colon and fecal concentrations of secondary bile acids in population samples from six countries. From (22).

associates point out, it need not be a highly potent agent to be important when an estimated *1300* grams of it is passed through the human colon over a 50-year period. In 1971, the same group reported the steroid concentrations in fecal samples from 127 persons in six countries of widely varying colon cancer incidence—England, Scotland, the United States, Uganda, Japan, and India—and showed a striking correlation (Fig. 3) between the average concentration of dihydroxycholanic acids (essentially a measure of deoxycholic acid) in these specimens and the incidence of colon cancer (22). Comparing fecal bacteria in the same population samples, they found larger numbers of anerobic organisms per unit weight of stool in the specimens from the United States and the United Kingdom than in those from Africa and Asia, and conversely smaller populations of aerobic species. These bacteriological findings may not be quite as significant as the data on bile acids, in the light of the very finicky growth requirements for isolating strict anerobic organisms; yet they are of special interest because of the greater capacity of anerobes to produce deoxycholic acid from cholic acid by 7-alpha dehydroxylation. Furthermore, within given bacterial species the *strains* isolated from the United States and British donors possessed this property more often than those from Asians and Africans. The donor groups from the high- and low-incidence countries were in fact known to be consuming the diets characteristic of those countries, except for a group of vegans residing in England and a group of English residents from Uganda who consumed a typical English diet. Taking into account the bacteriological findings in these subgroups, it was concluded that fecal flora were influenced much less by geography than by diet, and that the principal determinants of the diet were the levels of fat and protein intake. Of related interest, Reddy and his associates have used fecal β-glucuronidase levels as a biochemical measure of the metabolic activity of anerobic organisms in the colon, and have demonstrated highly significant increases in these levels in human volunteers ingesting a high-meat diet (23).

Is there a role for dietary fiber in this interaction of bacteria and bile salts? The stronger correlation of cancer prevalence with dietary fat, and of fecal anerobic bacteria with dietary fat, than with dietary fiber would suggest a negative answer, and no evidence has been found of a direct effect of dietary fiber on the composition of the fecal flora. To the extent, however, that fecal stasis may be favored in Western populations by fiber-deficient diets, both the concentration of and the duration of exposure to an intraluminal carcinogen would be increased. Furthermore, bile acids are known to be *absorbed* on fiber residues, and the possibility has been raised that they might thus be protected from the action of dehydroxylating enzymes in gut bacteria. Pomare and Heaton (Table 8) recently reported that feeding bran to subjects with intact gall bladders reduced the proportion of deoxycholate in the bile salt pool, while increasing the proportion of chenodeoxycholate (24). Since these changes are quite significant and were achieved with "physiological" amounts of bran (that is, 30 g/day, or the equivalent of the fiber content of 165 g of whole wheat flour) and were demonstrable after only 6 to 10 weeks, the role of dietary fiber as a lifelong determinant of bile salt metabolism may indeed be quite important. If present notions about the carcinogenicity of the secondary bile acids are correct, the deficiency of fiber in the American diet may bear a portion of the blame for the high prevalence of cancer of the colon.

Cholelithiasis (Gallstones)

Much of the evidence just presented can be viewed as potentially important in the etiology of cholelithiasis. Although undoubtedly be-

Table 8   Effect of Bran on Composition of Bile Salt Pool[a]

	Cholate (%)	Deoxycholate (%)	Chenodeoxycholate (%)
Control	42.2	27.1 ± 8.9	30.6 ± 3.6
Bran	42.2	13.8 ± 4.2	43.9 ± 2.7
p	N.S.	< 0.025	< 0.005

[a] Data from (24).

gun in early to middle life and then more common among women, the formation of gallstones continues and produces most of its serious and its lethal complications in the elderly. Beyond the age of 50, the two sexes are almost equally affected.

Seven years ago the chemical processes leading to the formation of gallstones in human beings were virtually unknown. Now, due in large measure to the work of Small (25) and Hofmann (26), we know that the common cholesterol stone precipitates in bile because the bile contains insufficient concentrations of bile acids and/or phospholipids to prevent oversaturation with cholesterol. The site of the metabolic abnormality has been identified as *not* the gall bladder *but* the hepatic parenchymal cell (27), and has been traced further to that cell's enzymatic mechanisms, which control the rates of cholesterol synthesis and of the formation of the bile acids, cholic and chenodeoxycholic acid ("cheno") from cholesterol. A key observation in establishing this point was that young women of certain American Indian tribes having an unusually high frequency of gallstones, though themselves not yet harboring such stones, secrete a "lithogenic bile" in which the concentration of "cheno" is abnormally low (28). The Mayo group has demonstrated in a small number of patients the partial or even complete dissolution of cholesterol gallstones in women *in vivo* by the prolonged feeding of "cheno," which leads to higher concentrations of this substance in the bile and enhanced solubility of cholesterol (29).

Though epidemiologic data on gallstone disease are not as abundant or as well founded as those for colonic cancer (30), its high frequency in the United States and Europe contrasts strikingly with numerous reports of its rarity in developing countries, and similar questions have been raised with respect to the possible etiologic role of the diet. It is noteworthy that all of the several models of cholesterol gallstone formation in experimental animals involve the feeding of semisynthetic diets containing large amounts of *refined* sugars and starches (31). Since some of the species used in these studies are accustomed to a high-carbohydrate diet, it is likely that the deprivation of the dietary fiber normally associated with carbohydrate intake is a significant factor.

Fiber deficiency in man leads to reduced synthesis of bile salts and decrease of their total concentration in bile; feeding of bran, on the other hand, reverses these effects. As indicated above, fiber deprivation appears to lead to a relative increase in the biliary concentration of deoxycholic acid by allowing bacterial dehydroxylation of cholic acid in the bowel (20). Conversely, the feeding of bran inhibits this process, and, in depressing the concentration of deoxycholic acid, removes its negative feedback effect on the production of chenodeoxycholic acid

(32), allowing the concentration of this compound to rise. Furthermore, "cheno" has been shown to inhibit the enzyme HMG Co-A reductase, which is rate-limiting in the synthesis of cholesterol by the liver. Thus bran, fed at levels that do not exceed the content of a natural diet, appears to mitigate or correct the abnormalities in biliary lipids believed to underlie the development of gallstones. Its effects qualitatively resemble those achieved by our present programs of feeding chenodeoxycholic acid in large doses.

COMMENT

A number of other gastrointestinal problems common to elderly persons have been thought to be aggravated or induced, albeit indirectly, by the American diet. The data on the association of these with our Western way of life are not adequate, and the theoretical basis for the most part is a simple one. Hemorrhoids and hiatal hernia may indeed be aggravated by the high intraabdominal pressure generated in passing small dry stools, but the evidence is limited and not convincing. It is probably true that acute appendicitis occurs less often in developing countries than in the United States, but this is not a major disease of the elderly, and the downward trend in incidence of appendicitis in our country would tend to dissociate it from the evidence implicating dietary factors in the causation of diverticular disease, colon cancer, and gallstones.

Those three diseases are extremely costly to the United States in terms of loss of life, of morbidity, and of the costs of health care. In 1967 the cost of surgery alone for the removal of diseased American gallbladders was estimated at half a billion dollars annually (33), with the added economic losses due to time away from the job and due to premature death being at least as large. A reasonable estimate of annual economic loss for these three diseases, including the costs of health care as well as losses in productivity due to morbidity and mortality would be five or six billion 1974 dollars.

To counter this, it would appear that a very substantial, even a very expensive, program of preventive medicine, if it might reduce the frequency of these diseases to a point even halfway between our present figures and those of developing countries, might well be a bargain. It would be scientifically preferable to delay such efforts until all reasonable controversies in this area are resolved; and when they are, the actions taken can be much better directed. But here, as in the consideration of the hazards of cigarette smoking, the action indicated by existing data is to alter a habit pattern toward a preexisting norm for which *no* compensating biological disadvantage is now apparent, unless, as suggested by Correa and associates (34) "hard (cereal) grains" should by abrading the gastric mucosa constitute one of the factors that explain the geographic differences in prevalence of gastric cancer.

The epidemiologic evidence at hand, the onset of these digestive disorders in middle age, their long presymptomatic course in most individuals, and their severe impact on the quality of life in the aged, would seem to offer an important opportunity for real benefits from health education. Can we influence the coffee-and-danish breakfast, the hamburger for lunch, the soft-drink guzzling, the ice-cream-and-cake habits of our countrymen? I know we have other reasons than the control of these digestive diseases for such efforts, but even for that purpose the prospective benefits are truly staggering.

REFERENCES

1. Cowgill, G. R. and Anderson, W. E. *JAMA* **98:**1866 (1932).
2. McCance, R. A., Prior, K. M., Widdowson, E. M. *Brit. J. Nutr.* **7:**98 (1953).
3. Findlay, J. M., Smith, A. N., Mitchell, W. D. et al. *Lancet* **1:**146 (1974).
4. Burkitt, D. P. *Cancer* **28:**3 (1971).
5. Burkitt, D. P., Walker, A. R. P., and Painter, N. S. *Lancet* **4:**1408 (1972).
6. Manousos, O. N., Truelove, S. C., and Lumsden, K. *Brit. Med. J.* **3:**762 (1967).
7. Kyle, J., Adesola, A. D., Tinckler, L. F., and deBeaux, J. *Scand. J. Gastroenterology* **2:**77 (1967).
8. Carlson, A. J. and Hoelzel, F. *Gastroenterology* **12:**108 (1949).
9. Wierda, J. L. *Arch. Path.* **36:**621 (1943).
10. Hodgson, W. J. B. *Gut* **13:**802 (1972).
11. Arfwidsson, S. *Acta. Chir. Scandinav.*, Suppl. 342, Stockholm, 1964.
12. Hodgson, J. *Brit. Med. J.* **3:**729 (1972).
13. Devroede, G. J. In *Fiber Deficiency and Colonic Disorders.* R. W. Reilly and J. B. Kirsner, Eds., Plenum, New York, 1975, pp. 120-123.
14. Painter, N. S., Almeida, A. Z., and Colebourne, K. W. *Brit. Med. J.* **1:**137, (1972).
15. Haenszel, W. and Correa, P. *Cancer* **28:**14 (1971).
16. Haenszel, W. *J. Nat. Cancer Inst.* **26:**37 (1961).
17. Haenszel, W. and Kurihara, M. *J. Nat. Cancer Inst.* **40:**43 (1968).
18. Drasar B. S. and Irving, D. *Brit. J. Cancer* **27:**167 (1973).
19. Weisburger, J. *Cancer* **28:**60 (1971).
20. Hill, M. J. *Cancer* **34:**815 (1974).
21. Hill, M. J., Drasar, B. S., Meade, T. W., et al. *Lancet* **1:**535 (1975).
22. Hill, M. J., Crowther, J. S., Drasar, B. S., et al. *Lancet* **1:**95 (1971).
23. Reddy, B. S., Weisburger, J. H., and Wynder, E. L. *Science* **183:**416 (1974.

24. Pomare, E. W. and Heaton, K. W. *Brit. Med. J.* **4:**262 (1973).

25. Small, D. M. *Adv. Intern. Med.* **16:**243, (1970).

26. Hofmann, A. F. and Small, D. M. *Ann. Rev. Med.* **18:**333 (1967).

27. Small, D. M. and Rapo, S. *New Engl. J. Med.* **283:**53 (1970).

28. Thistle, J. L. and Schoenfield, L. J. *New Engl. J. Med.* **284:**177 (1971).

29. Danzinger, R. G., Hofmann, A. F., Schoenfield, L. J., and Thistle, J. L. *New Engl. J. Med.* **286:**1 (1972).

30. Kaye, M. D. and Kern, F. *Lancet* **2:**1228 (1971).

31. Dam, H. *Am. J. Med.* **51:**596 (1971).

32. Low-Beer, T. S. and Pomare, E. W. *Gastroenterology* **64:**764 (1973).

33. *A white paper by the American Gastroenterological Association, 1967. Gastroenterology* **53:**821, 1967.

34. Correa, P. Haenszel, W., Cuello, C. et al. *Lancet* **2:**58 (1975).

10

Obesity, Carbohydrate, and Lipid Interactions in the Elderly

EDWIN L. BIERMAN, M.D.

Head, Division of Metabolism and Gerontology, Professor of Medicine, University of Washington, Seattle, Washington

This chapter deals in general with fuel metabolism in man; specifically, with the role of obesity and aging, and their interaction, on the major fuels in the body—carbohydrates and lipids. A variety of changes in fuel metabolism occur with aging; some are related to intrinsic aging in the body and others are related to environmental factors that are in themselves related to age. What emerges and deserves particular emphasis is the course of events related to obesity.

If one considers over-all basal energy metabolism of the body (a composite of all fuel metabolism) it appears that after adulthood is reached there is a very gradual decline in basal energy metabolism in terms of oxygen consumption per square meter of body surface related to age (1). However, if one examines this slow decline in over-all body energy metabolism with age and considers it in terms of the body tissues that are actually doing the metabolizing, namely lean body mass, this slight decline is really not a decline at all, since there is a parallel change in body composition with age. A healthy 25-year-old man is not the same as a healthy 75-year-old man. His body composition has been changed. With aging, there is an increased proportion of adipose tissue at the expense of lean body mass (muscle tissue and bone) (2). The decline in bone mass with age has been discussed in Chapter 7. There is also a decline with age in muscle mass, which makes up the major fraction of lean body mass. This decline in muscle and bone is reflected by a gradual decrease in total body potassium with age (3). Thus, when one considers over-all energy metabolism again in terms of lean body

171

mass, since they both decline slowly at the same rate, there is no major decrease in intrinsic energy metabolism with aging.

However, as a result of this change in lean body mass, calorie requirements do change with aging. This is documented in data that were obtained in studies on a metabolic ward by Dr. Ahrens using constant composition liquid formula diets given in quantities necessary to maintain body weight (4). Retrospectively he analyzed how many calories were required to maintain constant weight in individuals of different ages. Among adult males and females, presumably because of this decline in lean body mass with age, there is a gradual decline in calorie requirements with age. The actual calculation of the regression equation suggests that there is a 43 calorie per decade decline in requirement for males and a 27 calorie per decade decline in requirements for females. Therefore there is a progressive decline in the need for calories with age, presumably as a result of this change in body composition. Of course many of us do not change our caloric intake with age despite this decline in requirement, so that there is a gradual buildup of fat tissue. The discussion about a change in body composition with an increase in relative adiposity assumes a constant body weight. However, in the real world, an individual's body weight does not remain constant throughout adult life. There have been a number of studies of populations at a given point in time (cross-sectional studies) which show that body weight in populations does change with age. In the Tecumseh study, a study of a population of about 10,000 individuals in Central Michigan, results show that in males there is a gradual increase in weight through adult life, reaching a peak in the middle years (about age 40 to 50), followed by a decline (5). In females, the same phenomenon is observed; however, the peak occurs about a decade later, at about age 50 to 60. Since these are cross-sectional studies, we do not know that an individual throughout life will follow this curve. In other words, if we follow a man throughout life would his weight follow this pattern? Only a longitudinal study would provide the answer. This might mean that, rather than the same individuals' gaining and losing weight throughout life, individuals who are the fattest are at the highest risk of early morbidity and mortality and they simply drop out of the population because of early death. Some insurance companies recognize the greater mortality risk of obesity by charging higher premiums for markedly overweight individuals.

It has become apparent from analysis of these age-related phenomena in terms of energy metabolism and body weight that the change in adiposity with age is probably more important in influencing the metabolic alterations observed with age than intrinsic changes in metabolic regulation caused by the aging process. In other words, environmental factors are probably more important with regard to age-related metabolic changes than intrinsic changes within the body. An example relates to blood glucose and carbohydrate metabolism.

In the Tecumseh study, and in other studies as well, blood glucose levels one hour after meals gradually increase with age in both males and females (6). This change in blood glucose with age is progressive. If one uses the standards of normality that usually apply in younger individuals, and applies them to the elderly population, one could conceivably make a diagnosis of diabetes in 50, 60, or even 80% of individuals over 65 years of age. In fact, this often occurs when hospital admissions of individuals over 65 years of age are analyzed. Many have "diabetes" by criteria that are developed in younger individuals. This phenomenon has been approached by Andres, who devised a nomogram for estimating blood glucose levels in terms of percentile rank, (where you stand with regard to your age peers) rather than in terms of a diagnosis (7). For example, a 25-year-old individual with a 2-hour blood glucose of 140 mg/100 ml, which is not unreasonable, will fall into the fourth or fifth percentile. This means that 95% of the population at age 25 have lower blood glucose levels and 5% higher, probably a good definition of upper limit of normal. But the same value for a 70-year-old man—140—is at the 50th percentile; half the population has higher and half the population lower blood glucose levels. Thus that level of blood glucose might be perfectly appropriate for an elderly individual.

This is not a phenomenon restricted to oral glucose tolerance. There is a progressive decline in the ability to handle intravenous glucose, probably as a result of the progressive decline in the early insulin response to the glucose challenge (8). This may well relate to obesity, since adiposity is associated with a certain resistance to insulin action in the tissues that metabolize fuels, mainly adipose tissue and muscle. As a result of this "insulin resistance," the pancreas responds by secreting more insulin, both in the basal state and after a glucose challenge. When obesity exists for many years, it puts stress on the insulin secretion mechanism, eventually unmasking those with genetic traits for diabetes (9). The same effect on insulin secretion may occur with aging. There is no way at present to distinguish the effects of aging on glucose metabolism from the effect of genetic diabetes. Thus adiposity existing for 10, 20, or 30 years will result in a progressive decline in the ability to respond to the glucose challenge with adequate insulin secretion and will lead to the progressive increase in blood glucose levels.

With regard to those factors related to lipid metabolism and aging in man, we shall focus on plasma cholesterol and plasma triglyceride, the two most important circulating lipids in terms of atherosclerosis, to be discussed by Goodman in the next chapter. Changes in lipid transport occur both in relation to age and in relation to obesity.

Serum cholesterol levels change with age. Again in data from the Tecumseh study (10), a gradual increase in cholesterol with age is observed in males up to the age of about 50, followed by a decline. With females an increase in cholesterol with age peaks about a decade later (age 60). The same problems exist in the analysis of this cross-sectional study as existed with body weight. Individuals with a higher cholesterol simply may have dropped out of the population because of earlier disease and death.

The same phenomenon is observed with serum triglyceride levels. In data obtained from over 2000 individuals in Stockholm (11), there is a gradual increase in plasma triglyceride levels with age, reaching a peak at age 45 to 50, followed by a decline. In females there is a gradual increase with age at lesser levels, again reaching a peak a decade later at age 55 to 60. We have observed the same phenomenon in Seattle (12). Results obtained in a large control population for a myocardial infarct study show that in males there is a gradual increase in cholesterol levels with age. There seems to be a peak at age 40 to 50, followed by a decline. In females the peak appears to be at age 60. With plasma triglycerides, peak levels are attained at age 40 to 50 in males and in females about a decade later. In a composite graph of serum cholesterol, serum triglyceride, and body weight plotted against age, the curves are superimposable (13). For males serum lipids and body weight peak at age 40 to 50 and in females a decade later at age 50 to 60. This strongly suggests that perhaps obesity or increasing adiposity with age is in some way responsible for these changes in serum lipids observed with age. It is of interest that neither serum lipids nor glucose increase with age in primitive people who remain thin throughout adulthood (14).

There are potential mechanisms whereby obesity might influence serum lipid levels. With regard to triglyceride levels, increased insulin may be important. Since obesity produces insulin antagonism in the glucose-metabolizing tissues such that the pancreas puts out more insulin, and since insulin is one of the factors perfusing the liver and increasing endogenous triglyceride synthesis, increased levels of triglycerides could result from obesity by this mechanism. Triglyceride in the basal state is produced mainly in the liver, and increased synthesis results in hypertriglyceridemia. There are several ways to show that obesity leads to hypertriglyceridemia. Obesity does result in higher insulin levels and higher insulin levels are associated with higher triglyceride levels. There is also a relation between body weight and plasma triglyceride levels. Albrink also demonstrated a relationship between triglyceride level and weight gain in adults (15). Normal men from age 30 to age 70 who gained more than 10 pounds in weight after age 25 had higher triglyceride levels than those who did not.

An even better example of this relationship comes from the study of experimental obesity by Sims and co-workers (16). They paid normally thin volunteers who were in a penitentiary to gain weight. Fat tissue increased, mainly around the trunk (middle age spread), similar to what is observed in adult life. This experiment showed what the cross-sectional studies of naturally occurring obesity showed—that is, with increasing weight gain there is an increase in insulin levels, an increase in triglyceride levels, and as discussed below, an increase in cholesterol levels.

As shown by Goodman and his colleagues (17), as well as by others (18), cholesterol production rates in man also increase with obesity.

In population data, the fattest individuals have higher cholesterol levels than the thinnest (10). This relationship is certainly true of males and is a little less well defined for females. In the Framingham study, a study of the whole population of a town in Massachusetts, various parameters were measured and then subjects were followed for more than 15 years. In the follow-up period there was a direct relationship between the amount of weight gained and the degree of rise in serum cholesterol (19). For those individuals who lost weight, the reverse relationship held.

Thus obesity plays a profound role in fuel metabolism in the body, in glucose, in cholesterol, and in triglyceride metabolism. Obesity does change with age as discussed. Another consequence of obesity, in addition to these changes in fuel metabolism, is its association with the age-related diseases diabetes and atherosclerosis. There is a possible relationship between obesity on the one hand and the development of diabetes and atherosclerosis, two prominent age-related metabolic diseases, on the other (13). Obesity results in insulin antagonism, high insulin levels, increased synthesis of triglyceride and cholesterol, high circulating lipoprotein levels, and ultimately lipid deposition in arteries and atherosclerosis. Insulin might also affect the metabolism of the arterial wall directly, thereby contributing to atherosclerosis. Obesity acting over many years ultimately leads to a diminished insulin secretion by the pancreas, producing at first glucose intolerance, then basal hyperglycemia, and ultimately clinical diabetes. As the diabetic state progresses, lipoprotein removal from the circulation is impaired, leading to further hyperlipidemia and enhancement of the atherosclerotic process.

In summary, both intrinsic body processes and, more important, environmental factors operating over many years, apparently act together with unknown genetic factors to produce a variety of changes in carbohydrate and lipid metabolism, resulting in these two highly prevalent age-related diseases—diabetes and atherosclerosis. The most prominent environmental factors during life may well be those producing increasing adiposity.

REFERENCES

1. Spector, W. S. *Handbook of Biological Data.* Saunders, Philadelphia, 1961.

2. Lesser, G. T., Kumar, I., and Steele, J. M. *Ann. N.Y. Acad. Sci.* **131:**559 (1965).

3. Allen, R. H., Anderson, E. C., and Langham, W. H. *J. Gerontol.* **15:**348 (1960).

4. Ahrens, E. H., Jr.: The use of liquid formula diets in metabolic studies: 15 years' experience. In *Advances in Metabolic Disorders, Vol. 4.* R. Levine and R. Luft, Eds., Academic, New York, 1970, pp. 297-332.

5. Montoye, H. J., Epstein, F. H., and Kjelsberg, M. O. *Am. J. Clin. Nutr.* **16:**417 (1965).

6. Hayner, N. S., Kjelsberg, M. O., Epstein, F. H., and Francis, T., Jr. *Diabetes* **14:**413, (1965).

7. Andres, R. *Mayo Clinic Proc.* **42:**413 (1967).

8. Crockford, P. M., Harbeck, R. J., and Williams, R. H. *Lancet* **2:**465 (1966).

9. Bierman, E. L., Bagdade, J. D., and Porte, D., Jr. *Amer. J. Clin. Nutr.* **21:**1434 (1968).

10. Montoye, H. J., Epstein, F. H., and Kjelsberg, M. O. *Amer. J. Clin. Nutr.* **18:**397, (1966).

11. Carlson, M. P. and Bottiger, E., *Lancet* **1:**865 (1972).

12. Goldstein, J. L., Hazzard, W. R., Schrott, H. G., Bierman, E. L., and Motulsky, A. G. *J. Clin. Invest.* **52:**1533 (1973).

13. Bierman, E. L. *Mech. Aging and Devel.* **2:**315 (1973).

14. Goldrick, R. B., Sinnett, P. F., and Whyte, H. M.: An assessment of coronary heart disease and coronary risk factors in a New Guinea highland population. In: *Atherosclerosis: Proceedings of the Second International Symposium.* R. J. Jones, Ed., Springer-Verlag, New York, 1970, pp. 366-68.

15. Albrink, M. J., Meigs, J. W., and Granoff, M. A. *New Eng. J. Med.* **266:**484 (1962).

16. Sims, E. A. H., Horton, E. S., and Salans, B. *Ann. Rev. Med.* **22:**235 (1971).

17. Nestel, P. J., Whyte, H. M., and Goodman, D. S. *J. Clin. Invest.* **48:**982 (1969).

18. Miettinen, T. A. *Circulation* **44:**842 (1971).

19. Kannel, W. B. *Nutrah* (Amer. Heart Assoc), **1**(3), 1-4 (1973).

11

Hyperlipidemia, Arteriosclerosis, and Ischemic Heart Disease

DeWITT S. GOODMAN and FRANK REES SMITH

Department of Medicine, Columbia University, College of Physicians and Surgeons, New York, New York

Cardiovascular diseases account for 53% of all deaths in the United States and cost the economy more than $20 billion per year in lost productivity and expenses for medical care, disability, and death (1). In our country in 1972 deaths from cardiovascular disease were approximately 3 times the rate of those from the second leading cause of death, cancer. The relative importance of cardiovascular disease, in terms of percent of all deaths for a given age group, rises steadily with age. Thus, while cardiovascular disease accounts for 28% of all deaths in the age group from 35 to 44 years, it accounts for 69% in the group 75 years and older (1). This reflects in part the continued progression with age of arteriosclerosis, the pathological process underlying the major form of heart disease (ischemic heart disease).

Epidemiological studies have shown that coronary arteriosclerotic heart disease occurs with increased frequency in association with certain characteristics present in the population under study, or in their environment. These characteristics have been termed risk factors. The major risk factors indicated by a variety of studies (2–8) conducted chiefly in the past two decades are elevated serum lipids, specifically cholesterol and probably triglycerides; hypertension; cigarette smoking; elevated blood sugar (diabetes mellitus); and personality factors (or certain patterns of behavior) (9). Other risk factors for which there is some evidence include obesity, sedentary living, and a family history of premature clinical atherosclerosis. It is possible on the basis of these risk factors to identify persons especially susceptible to the develop-

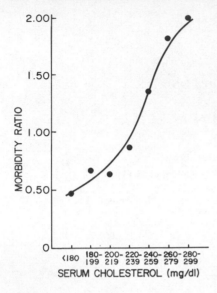

Figure 1. Risk of coronary heart disease during 14-year follow-up in the Framingham study (3) for men age 30 to 49 at entry as plotted against serum cholesterol level at initial examination. Morbidity ratio incidence rate for coronary heart disease for each subgroup divided by incidence rate for total population of Framingham men this age.

ment of the clinical complications of atherosclerosis, and to develop programs of primary prevention.

Prospective epidemiological studies have provided detailed quantitative information about the relationship between the serum cholesterol concentration and the statistical risk of developing ischemic heart disease. Figure 1 shows this relationship as determined in the study conducted in Framingham, Massachusetts (3). The data demonstrate that there is a continuous relationship between the level of serum cholesterol and coronary risk: risk rises continuously throughout a wide range of cholesterol levels, and not just in people with clearly elevated levels of cholesterol. Nutritional factors play an important role in influencing the serum cholesterol concentration and hence the level of coronary risk. Thus, epidemiological studies in a variety of populations have related the type of diet eaten both to plasma cholesterol concentration and to the frequency of coronary heart disease (10, 11).

The effects of the major risk factors are roughly additive, so that persons with multiple risk factors have a greatly increased risk of developing clinical coronary heart disease. Table 1, taken from the Framingham data (12), illustrates the interplay between serum cholesterol concentration and systolic blood pressure. The 6-year probability for developing coronary heart disease in a 45-year-old man is shown in terms of the cholesterol level and systolic blood pressure as variables. At the lowest cholesterol concentration (185 mg/dl) and systolic blood pressure (105 mm Hg) the probability is 1.5%, whereas at the highest

Table 1   Probability (in percent) of a 45-year-old Man's Developing Coronary Heart Disease in 6 Years[a]

Serum Cholesterol (mg/dl)	Systolic Blood Pressures (mm Hg)						
	105	120	135	150	165	180	195
185	1.5	1.8	2.1	2.5	3.1	3.7	4.4
210	1.9	2.2	2.7	3.2	3.9	4.6	5.5
235	2.4	2.9	3.4	4.1	4.9	5.9	7.0
260	3.0	3.6	4.3	5.2	6.2	7.4	8.7
285	3.8	4.6	5.5	6.5	7.8	9.2	10.9
310	4.9	5.8	6.9	8.2	9.8	11.5	13.6
335	6.2	7.3	8.7	10.3	12.2	14.3	16.7

[a] Assuming that he does not smoke cigarettes, does not have glucose intolerance or left ventricular hypertrophy by electrocardiogram. The values are derived from the Framingham data (12).

values shown (cholesterol of 335 mg/dl and systolic blood pressure of 195 mm Hg) the probability rises to 16.7%. Moreover, for each level of serum cholesterol and blood pressure a cigarette smoker has a higher risk than a nonsmoker.

Serum triglyceride concentrations also appear to have an important quantitative relationship to the probability of developing coronary heart disease. Studies by Albrink, Meigs, and Man (13), and by Goldstein and co-workers (14) implicate hypertriglyceridemia in the etiology of ischemic heart disease. Furthermore, the prospective study of males in Stockholm (8) suggests that serum cholesterol and triglyceride concentrations operate independently as risk factors.

It is difficult to determine acceptable "normal" limits for serum cholesterol and triglyceride concentrations. In addition to the phenomenon of continuously rising risk one must deal with the problem of the increase in serum concentrations of cholesterol and triglycerides as the population becomes older. The mean concentrations and deviations of serum cholesterol in 1492 men from 20 to 70 years of age (7) are shown in Figure 2. Mean concentrations increase from 160 to 170 mg/dl in the population in their 20s to a level of 250 to 260 in the fifth decade, before declining thereafter. The decline in cholesterol concentrations in the older age groups may reflect the higher death rate and

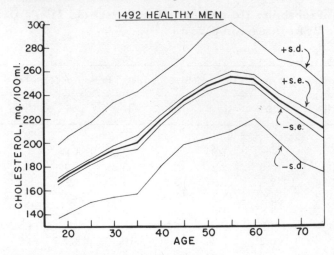

Figure 2.   Change in serum cholesterol concentration with age in men from (7).

earlier death of younger individuals with high cholesterol concentrations. One approach to the problem of determining which values should be considered abnormal has been to determine the serum cholesterol and triglyceride concentrations that separate the upper 5% of the population from the lower 95% (the 95th percentile values). The values currently used by the Center for Prevention of Premature Arteriosclerosis in New York City (see below) as 95th percentile estimates for serum cholesterol levels in men are 260, 270, 280, and 290 mg/dl for ages 21 to 29, 30 to 39, 40 to 49, and 50 to 59, respectively. Estimates of the 95th percentile values for fasting triglyceride levels have been reported by Levy and colleagues (15) as 140, 150, 160, and 190 mg/dl for the same four age groups. Values above the 95th percentile are considered clearly elevated, and hence are defined as hyperlipidemic.

Hyperlipidemia is a particularly prominent finding among young people who develop clinical ischemic heart disease. Figure 3 shows the relationship between age and sex and frequency of hyperlipidemia in 500 survivors of myocardial infarction, reported from Seattle (14). Hyperlipidemia was arbitrarily defined as cholesterol and/or triglyceride values exceeding the 95th percentile for the control group (spouse controls of infarct survivors). A very high frequency of hyperlipidemia (60%) was found in male survivors less than 40 years old and in female survivors below age 50. While the frequency of hyperlipidemia decreased in males as age increased, hyperlipidemia was found at rela-

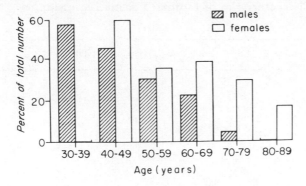

Figure 3. Relation between frequency of hyperlipidemia and age and sex of survivors of myocardial infarction in the Seattle study (14).

tively high frequencies in women in all age groups. It has been suggested that the relatively low frequency of hyperlipidemia (as defined here) in older men developing ischemic heart disease may reflect the fact that the "normal" lipid values in our population are really too high (in absolute terms), and hence predispose to a high rate of disease in the general population. While this may well be the case, we should also remember that the development of atherosclerosis is a multifactorial process, involving an interplay of many environmental as well as genetic factors.

Lipids are not soluble in water; they circulate in plasma in association with certain specific proteins in the form of plasma lipoproteins. Four classes of specific lipoproteins circulate in plasma, and the characteristics of these are summarized in Table 2. Two of these, chylomicrons and very-low-density lipoproteins (VLDL), are composed predominantly of triglyceride, and represent, respectively, the transport form of exogenous (dietary) and of endogenous triglyceride. The low-density, or β-lipoprotein, contains cholesterol as its major component, and normally represents the circulating form of most of the plasma cholesterol. The chemistry and metabolism of the lipoproteins have been the subjects of intensive research activity in many laboratories during the past few years, and a great deal of information is being amassed about these interesting macromolecules.

The distribution of lipoproteins seen after serum is subjected to electrophoresis on paper or agarose gel was the basis of a system of classification for hyperlipidemia proposed by Fredrickson, Levy, and Lees (17). This typing system, as adopted by the World Health Organization (18), divided serum lipid disorders (elevations) into six types (I, IIa, IIb, III, IV, and V) depending on which lipoproteins were ele-

Table 2   Characteristics of Human Plasma Lipoproteins[a]

	Chylomicrons	VLDL[b]	LDL	HDL
Density	<1.006	<1.006	1.019–1.063	1.063–1.21
Electrophoretic mobility	(Origin)[c]	Pre-β	β	α
Size (diameter, nm)	75-200	30-80	20	7-10
Percent Composition				
Protein	2	10	25	50
Triglyceride	88	60	10	5
Cholesterol	5	12	50	20
Phospholipid	5	18	15	25

[a]Modified from (16). The % compositions are approximations.
[b]VLDL, Very low density lipoproteins; LDL, low density lipoproteins; HDL, high density lipoproteins.
[c]Chylomicrons remain at the origin on paper or agarose gel electrophoresis.

vated. The hyperlipoproteinemias commonly observed are type IIa (hyperbetalipoproteinemia, and hence hypercholesterolemia); type IIb (hyperbetalipoproteinemia plus hyperprebetalipoproteinemia, and hence hypercholesterolemia plus hypertriglyceridemia); and type IV (hyperprebetalipoproteinemia, and hence endogenous hypertriglyceridemia). Each of these three types was felt to be associated with an increase in incidence of arteriosclerosis.

Although the typing on the basis of lipoprotein electrophoresis does give a phenotypic description of the lipoprotein pattern at the time of sampling, recent family and genetic studies (19–22) suggest that lipoprotein phenotyping may have limited, if any, usefulness in the clinical management of patients with hyperlipidemia. Hazzard and his colleagues (19) in Seattle evaluated the lipoprotein phenotyping system in conjunction with a genetic study of 156 hyperlipidemia survivors of acute myocardial infarction. Lipoprotein phenotypes were compared with genetic analysis based on serum cholesterol and triglyceride concentrations in first- and second-degree relatives of survivors with hyperlipidemia. On an individual basis no lipoprotein pattern (among the types studied, which were IIa, IIb, IV, and V) proved to be specific for any particular genetic lipid disorder. Furthermore, no genetic disorder was specified by any one of these lipoprotein patterns. Hence the lipoprotein patterns presumably do not provide a classification according to specific pathogenetic defects.

Fasting total serum cholesterol and triglyceride concentrations alone have proved useful in genetic studies. In the Seattle study cited above (14, 20), the relatives of hyperlipidemic survivors of myocardial infarction were examined in detail. The majority of the hyperlipidemic survivors appeared to have genetic abnormalities, and in fact 54% were classified as having one of three conditions consistent with a monogenic pattern of inheritance. The most common genetic abnormality (30%) was familial combined hyperlipidemia, in which family members had elevated serum levels of either cholesterol or triglyceride or both. Familial hypertriglyceridemia was found in 14% of the hyperlipidemic survivors, and familial hypercholesterolemia was found in 10%.

In a study of 412 first-degree relatives of 101 survivors of myocardial infarction in Finland, Nikkilä and Aro (22) identified a familial trait in one-third of their survivors. As in the Seattle study, the combined disorder of cholesterol and triglyceride abnormalities was more common than either hypercholesterolemia or hypertriglyceridemia alone.

The practical conclusion from these studies is that in order to diagnose genetic disease it is necessary—since we lack specific genetic markers for the several conditions—to measure cholesterol and triglyceride concentrations of the first-degree relatives of an individual with hyperlipidemia. This offers families the benefit of having younger members with hyperlipidemia identified before they have symptomatic ischemic heart disease. Diagnosing genetic hyperlipidemia may also have prognostic value. In familial hypercholesterolemia Slack (23) calculated that the chance of a first attack of ischemic heart disease in males was 5.4% by the age of 30, 51% by age 50, and 85% by age 60. For women the risks were lower, at 0, 12%, and 57%, respectively. Stone and coworkers (24) showed a similar cumulative probability of ischemic heart disease of 16% in males with familial hypercholesterolemia at age 40 years, with a rise to 52% by age 60. As in Slack's study the risk was lower in females, lagging 20 years behind the risk in males. Familial hyperlipidemic individuals, then, merit maximum intervention therapy. It has been estimated that about 1 in 150 individuals in the general population may be a carrier of a gene predisposing to one of the three major familial lipid disorders.

One public health approach to the problem of the primary prevention of atherosclerosis and its complications (particularly ischemic heart disease) is to try to identify persons at high risk of coronary heart disease, and to enroll them in intervention programs designed to reduce this risk. The detection and diagnosis of hyperlipidemia is begun by a primary screening procedure, which usually consists of the measurement of serum cholesterol and triglyceride levels after an overnight fast. Such a primary screening for hyperlipidemia should be included as part of all periodic health examinations. If an elevated level (above the age-adjusted 95th percentile value) is found, a secondary screening procedure is undertaken, which consists first of confirming the presence of hyperlipidemia by repeating the laboratory analysis of fasting serum of plasma. When triglycerides are elevated, the presence of chylomicrons is sought by examining the sample after it has been in the refrigerator overnight, or by lipoprotein electrophoresis. Chylomicrons are normally absent in fasting serum. If hyperlipidemia is definitely present, then the possibility of its being secondary to some other disorder should be considered. Clinical studies should thus be conducted to rule out the causes of secondary hyperlipidemia (see Table 3) by history, physical examination, and appropriate laboratory tests. This is important, since the treatment of hyperlipidemia in patients with any of these conditions is first the treatment of the underlying primary disease or condition. In addition, a complete secondary screening procedure for patients with hyperlipidemia would include special laboratory tests if indicated (e.g., ultracentrifugation of plasma

Table 3

Hyperlipidemia may be secondary to

---

1. Obesity
2. Alcohol
3. Diabetes mellitus
4. Hypothyroidism
5. Chronic renal disease
6. Obstructive liver disease
7. Chronic pancreatitis
8. Dysglobulinemia — autoimmune disease
9. Oral contraceptives
10. Pregnancy
11. Glucocorticoid excess
12. Porphyria
13. Other causes

---

for the diagnosis of the type III disorder), and the study of family members for genetic analysis.

In summary, then, the study of patients with hyperlipidemia should proceed in four stages: (*1*) description of the lipid (and lipoprotein) abnormality; (*2*) analysis of etiology (primary vs. secondary disorder); (*3*) identification of familial status (familial vs. nonfamilial); and (*4*) management.

Treatment of hyperlipidemia is based on the assumption that the lowering of the coronary risk factor (elevated serum cholesterol or triglyceride level) will result in a commensurate lowering of coronary risk itself. Definitive evidence that changing a coronary risk factor will reduce coronary risk is available only for the case of cigarette smoking. Thus, the Framingham study has shown that people who stop smoking have a coronary risk close to that of people who never smoked. For the factor of hyperlipidemia, however, such proof is not now available, although large-scale clinical trials are in progress aimed at trying to obtain such evidence.

Management of hyperlipidemia first involves modifying the diet so as to lower serum cholesterol and/or triglyceride level. Epidemiologic data have given rise to the attractive hypothesis that lowering serum cholesterol by diet may retard the development of atherosclerosis and its complications (25). Definitive testing of this important hypothesis in humans would require mass field trials using a relatively young, healthy population requiring 8,000 to 219,000 subjects, depending on the design of the study (26). Such an extensive diet–heart study has not been undertaken largely because of the enormous costs involved, but smaller studies testing the diet hypothesis have been undertaken. Experimental subjects on a low-cholesterol, low saturated fat, higher polyunsaturated fat diet have been compared with control subjects by Dayton and colleagues over 8 years using domiciled veterans (27), by Leren over 11 years using men in Oslo after an initial myocardial infarction (28), and by Miettinen and colleagues over 12 years using a crossover design involving the inhabitants of two mental hospitals in Helsinki (29). The results of these studies suggest that lowering the serum cholesterol concentration by dietary means will lower the incidence of new events of coronary heart disease. Further suggestive evidence is available from private studies in which dietary manipulation has produced regression of coronary atheromatosis in rhesus monkeys (30).

Taken together, the evidence from these and other studies strongly suggests that modifying the diet to lower serum cholesterol level is desirable in people with high lipid levels or with elevated coronary risk due to other risk factors, and perhaps in the general population as well. This is particularly true for people with clear-cut hyperlipidemia (> 95th percentile values). Many patients will show substantial (20% or more) reductions in serum lipid levels in response to diet. Many patients will, however, remain hyperlipidemic despite dietary therapy, and in these patients the question of the desirability of drug treatment to lower serum lipid levels must then be considered.

It is often difficult to decide whether a given patient warrants treatment with lipid-lowering drugs. In general, we currently believe that the benefit/risk ratio is high enough in the high-risk patients (lipid values above the 95th percentile) to warrant such treatment. This is particularly true for those patients who manifest other risk factors in addition to hyperlipidemia, or who have familial hyperlipidemia. Clinical trials designed to evaluate the effectiveness of treatment in reducing coronary risk are currently being introduced or are underway. One of these, an ongoing study by Oliver and his colleagues, being conducted in Edinburgh, Prague, and Budapest, is a primary prevention trial using clofibrate to lower hyperlipidemia in men age 30 to 59 (31). Another study, which has been in progress for several years and is just being completed, is the Coronary Drug Project (CDP) (32–34).). This project, a nationwide collaborative project sponsored by the National Heart and Lung Institute, is a secondary prevention study in men age 30 to 64 years with proven previous myocardial infarction. Of the four drugs studied in the CDP, two (conjugated estrogens and dextrothyroxine) have been discontinued for undesirable effects, and two (clofibrate and nicotinic acid) have been continued to the end of the study. Two other major collaborative (multiclinic) primary prevention trials are being introduced in this country. One of these is the Lipid Research Clinics' trial of cholestyramine resin in type II hyperlipoproteinemic men. The other is the Multiple Risk Factor Intervention Trial (MRFIT), which will assess the effectiveness of measures to reduce elevated serum cholesterol (by diet), high blood pressure (by diet and drugs), and cigarette smoking. It is hoped that these studies will in time provide definitive evidence that intervention programs directed at known coronary risk factors, and specifically at hyperlipidemia, can indeed reduce coronary risk.

In New York City we are engaged in a collaborative research program, the Center for Prevention of Premature Arteriosclerosis (CPPA), involving investigators and clinicians at Rockefeller University, Columbia University's College of Physicians and Surgeons, and the Albert Einstein College of Medicine. The CPPA is developing a clinical trial to determine whether clofibrate or cholestyramine resin, or the two drugs together, are more desirable than diet alone in the treatment of patients with various kinds of primary hyperlipidemia who are otherwise well. "Desirability" will be assessed mainly by plasma lipid responses, patient adherence, and the lack of drug toxicity or side effects. In addition, other clinical and metabolic studies dealing with various aspects of hyperlipidemia, arteriosclerosis, and coronary heart disease are in progress in this Center.

The plasma cholesterol concentration is influenced by the amount of cholesterol in the diet, and also by the amounts of saturated and polyunsaturated fat in the diet. In one study, Mattson and his colleagues (35) fed increasing amounts of cholesterol to human volunteers, and found consistent dose-related increases in serum cholesterol levels. Moreover, Connor and co-workers (36) have shown that the effect of dietary cholesterol is independent of that of dietary fat. Thus, subjects on a cholesterol-free intake showed a fall in serum cholesterol level in spite of a high intake of saturated fat, whereas subjects given a high cholesterol intake showed an increase in serum cholesterol level in spite of a high intake of polyunsaturated fat. Numerous studies (37, 38) have shown that polyunsaturated fat has a hypocholesterolemic effect, whereas saturated fats in the diet have an opposite effect.

Based on these and other observations, our approach to dietary therapy involves the use of a diet limited in cholesterol and saturated animal fat, with caloric intake appropriate for the patient to achieve and maintain an ideal body weight. Weight reduction is stressed in overweight patients, particularly in those with hypertriglyceridemia. The diet that we have found most useful has been described in detail by the American Heart Association (39). Dietary cholesterol is limited to less than 300 mg/day, the fat content to 35% of total calories, and the saturated fat to less than 10% of calories. In practical terms the diet limits egg consumption to two per week, eliminates butter, cream, and whole milk, and emphasizes fruits, vegetables, polyunsaturated margarines, lean meat, chicken, and fish. With such a diet one can anticipate a 10 to 20% reduction in serum cholesterol concentration (40, 41). Studies conducted with this diet have also demonstrated reductions in serum triglyceride concentration (40, 42), particularly in patients who are both hypertriglyceridemic and obese. In a series of such men, Hall and co-workers observed an average reduction of serum triglycerides of 17%, along with a 12% reduction in serum cholesterol levels and a 5.3% decrease in body weight (42). It was concluded (42) that "a low carbohydrate diet is seldom required to achieve significant lowering of serum triglyceride in middle-aged, obese, hypertriglyceridemic men, with or without hypercholesterolemia, providing that weight loss is accomplished and sustained, and intake of saturated fat and cholesterol is low."

In those individuals who remain hyperlipidemic after perhaps 6 months on the above diet it is appropriate to consider the use of medication. Currently clofibrate and bile-sequestering resin such as cholestyramine are the drugs of choice. Clofibrate appears to be more effective in hypertriglyceridemia, whereas cholestyramine resin is emphasized in hypercholesterolemia. Both drugs may be required in some patients with hypertriglyceridemia and hypercholesterolemia.

Arteriosclerosis and its cardiovascular complications, particularly ischemic heart disease, are phenomena that seem clearly tied to the aging process in humans. The aim of preventive therapy is to retard or prevent the progression of the atherosclerotic process and the appearance of clinical disease. Our best approach at this time is intervention directed at the known major coronary risk factors. A judicious diet low in cholesterol and saturated fat, and the achievement and maintenance of an ideal body weight, are the keystone of current intervention therapy for the risk factor of hyperlipidemia.

REFERENCES

1. American Heart Association. *Heart Facts 1975*. New York, 1974.

2. Kannel, W. B., Dawber, T. R., Kagan, A., Revotskie, N., and Stokes, J. III. *Ann. Int. Med.* **55**:33 (1961).

3. Kannel, W. B., Castelli, W. P., Gordon, T., and McNamara, P. M. *Ann. Int. Med.* **74**:1 (1971).

4. Leren, P. *Acta Med. Scand.* **466**:Supplement I, 1 (1966).

5. Epstein, F. H. *J. Chronic Dis.* **18**:735 (1965).

6. Deutscher, S., Epstein, F. H., and Keller, J. B. *Am. J. Epid.* **89**:510 (1969).

7. Stamler, J., Berkson, D. M., Lindberg, H. A., Hall, Y., Miller, W., et al. *Med. Clin. N. Am.* **50**:229 (1966).

8. Carlson, L. A. and Böttiger, *Lancet* **1**:865 (1972).

9. Jenkins, C. D. *New Eng. J. Med.* **284**:244, 307 (1971).

10. Keys, A., Anderson, J. T., Aresu, M., Biorck, G., Brock, J. F., et al. *J. Clin. Invest.* **35**:1173 (1956).

11. Keys, A., Kimura, N., Kusukawa, A., Bronte-Stewart, B., Larsen, N., and Keys, M. H. *Ann. Int. Med.* **48**:83 (1958).

12. American Heart Association. Coronary Risk Handbook—Estimating Risk of Coronary Heart Disease in Daily Practice. New York, 1973.

13. Albrink, M. J., Meigs, J. W., and Man, E. B. *Am. J. Med.* **31**:4 (1961).

14. Goldstein, J. L., Hazzard, W. R., Bierman, E. L., Schrott, H. G., and Motulsky, A. G. *J. Clin. Invest.* **52**:1533 (1973).

15. Levy, R. I., Fredrickson, D. S., Shulman, R., Bilheimer, D. W., Breslow, J. L., et al. *Ann. Int. Med.* **77**:267 (1972).

16. Levy, R. I., Morganroth J., and Rifkind, B. M. *New Eng. J. Med.* **290:**1295 (1974).

17. Fredrickson, D. S., Levy, R. I., and Lees, R. S. *New Eng. J. Med.* **276:**32, 94, 148, 215, 273 (1967).

18. Beaumont, J. L., Carlson, L. A., Cooper, G. R., Fejfar, Z., Fredrickson, D. S., and Strasser, T. *Bull Wld. Hlth. Org.* **43:**891 (1970).

19. Hazzard, W. R., Goldstein, J. L., Schrott, H. G., Motulsky, A. G., and Bierman, E. L. *J. Clin. Invest.* **52:**1569 (1973).

20. Goldstein, J. L., Schrott, H. G., Hazzard, W. R., Bierman E. L., and Motulsky, A. G. *J. Clin. Invest.* **52:**1544 (1973).

21. Rose, H. G., Kranz, P., Weinstock, M., Juliano, J., and Haft, J. I. *Am. J. Med.* **54:**148 (1973).

22. Nikkilä, E. A. and Aro, A. *Lancet* **1:**954 (1973).

23. Slack, J. *Lancet* **2:**1380 (1969).

24. Stone, N. J., Levy, R. I., Fredrickson, D. S., and Verter, J. *Circulation* **49:**476 (1974).

25. Connor, W. E. and Connor, S. L. *Prev. Med.* **1:**49 (1972).

26. Mass Field Trials of the Diet-Heart Question. Their Significance, Timeliness, Feasibility and Applicability. Report of the Diet-Heart Panel of the National Heart Institute, E. H. Ahrens, Jr., Chairman. American Heart Association Monograph Number 28. American Heart Association, Inc. New York, 1969.

27. Dayton, S., Pierce, M. L., Hashimoto, S., Dixon, W. J., and Tomiyasu, U. *Circulation* **40:**Supplement II, 1 (1969).

28. Leren, P. *Circulation* **42:**935 (1970).

29. Miettinen, M., Karvonen, M. J., Turpeinen, O., Elosuo, R., and Paavilainen, E. *Lancet* **2:**835 (1972).

30. Armstrong, M. L., Warner, E. D., and Connor, W. E. *Circ. Res.* **27:**59 (1970).

31. Oliver, M. F. A primary prevention trial using clofibrate to lower hyperlipidemia. In *Atheroschlerosis.* R. J. Jones, Ed., Springer-Verlag, New York, 1970, pp. 582-586.

32. Coronary Drug Project Research Group. *Circulation* **47:**Supplement I, 1 (1973).

33. Coronary Drug Project Research Group. *J. A. M. A.* **220:**996 (1972).

34. Coronary Drug Project Research Group. *J. A. M. A.* **226:**652 (1973).

35. Mattson, F. H., Erickson, B. A., and Kligman, A. M. *Am. J. Clin. Nutr.* **25:**589 (1972).

36. Connor, W. E., Stone, D. B., and Hodges, R. E. *J. Clin. Invest.* **43:**1691 (1964).

37. Ahrens, E. H., Jr., Hirsch, J., Insull, W., Jr., Tsaltas, T. T., Blomstrand, R., and Peterson, M. L. *Lancet* **1:**943 (1957).

38. Keys, A., Anderson, J. T., and Grande, F. *Lancet* **2:**959 (1957).

39. American Heart Association, Committee on Nutrition, *Diet and Coronary Heart Disease* New York, 1973.

40. Wilson, W. S., Hulley, S. B., Burrows, M. I., and Nichaman, M. Z. *Am. J. Med.* **51:**491 (1971).

41. Lees, R. S. and Wilson, D. E. *New Eng. J. Med.* **284:**186 (1971).

42. Hall, Y., Stamler J., Cohen, D. B., Majonnier, L., Epstein, M. B., et al. *Atherosclerosis* **16:**389 (1972).

Index